OLD-AGE POLITICS IN CALIFORNIA

OLD-AGE POLITICS IN CALIFORNIA

FROM RICHARDSON TO REAGAN

JACKSON K. PUTNAM

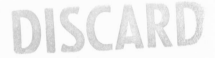

STANFORD UNIVERSITY PRESS
STANFORD, CALIFORNIA
1970

Sources of photos and illustrations:
Nos. 1, 2, 4–6, 9–11, 13, 15, 17, 18, United Press International Photos
No. 3, courtesy of the *San Francisco Examiner*
Nos. 7, 8, 12, 14, 16, Wide World Photos

Preface

Writing on the subject of old-age politics is not the easiest of tasks for the historian. Most historians ignore the subject entirely or treat it superficially as either an aberrant curiosity or a natural component of the depression syndrome of the 1930's. That the problems of aging in modern society are cultural, social, and psychological as well as economic seems largely to have escaped them. Behavioral scientists, for their part, have studied many aspects of the problem of aging with great sophistication and insight, and have produced a rich and voluminous literature on gerontology and geriatrics. But unfortunately, their studies, like many others of this type, are radically "presentist" in scope, and lacking in any real historical dimension. They shed little light on how the conditions they describe and analyze came about over a given period of time; nor is there a sense of the development of an old-age political movement arising out of these conditions and gathering momentum with their persistence.

In this book I have tried to right the balance somewhat by tracing the development of an old-age political movement in a single state in a rather traditional historical fashion, and at the same time drawing on the findings of behavioral scientists to interpret the historical events reported. I see this study as only explorative, as simply a modest beginning; much more can and needs to be said on the subject of old-age politics in California.

I am deeply in debt to many persons for their assistance in the preparation of this book, indeed too many to name here. To a few, however, I must express my great gratitude. Don E. Fehrenbacher of Stanford University saw the manuscript through the

Ph.D. dissertation phase and, more, assisted me in finding a publisher. His colleague Thomas A. Bailey also read the original manuscript and contributed greatly to whatever stylistic merit it possesses. Andrew F. Rolle of Occidental College gave much encouragement and assistance in securing publication, and J. G. Bell and Ellen Pulfrey of Stanford University Press have been extraordinarily helpful in editing and otherwise improving the quality of the finished work. Finally, my wife, Patricia Harris Putnam, not only assisted in the proofreading but also gracefully accepted her role of "research widow," and both created and preserved that relaxed and congenial home atmosphere so necessary for the completion of any sustained effort.

Needless to say, none of the aforementioned are in any way responsible for the errors and shortcomings in this book. I cheerfully accept that responsibility for myself.

J.K.P.

California State College
Fullerton

Contents

Eight pages of photographs follow p. 102

OLD-AGE POLITICS IN CALIFORNIA

1

The Problems of the Aged

IN THE twentieth century California's population has changed in four major ways: it has grown very large; it has become highly urbanized; it has settled increasingly in the southern part of the state; and it has "aged." From about one-and-one-half million at the turn of the century, California's population has grown to an estimated twenty million in 1969, and the state is now generally recognized as the most populous in the nation. The vast majority of California's inhabitants live in cities; by 1960 the state was 86.4 per cent urban, a percentage exceeded only by New Jersey.[1] Likewise a growing majority have chosen to live in the southern eight counties of the state, particularly in the mushrooming Los Angeles area. Only a "cow county" in the 1880's, Los Angeles contained 20 per cent of the state's total population in 1900, 39 per cent in 1920, 53 per cent in 1940, and probably close to 60 per cent in 1969.[2]

Of greater importance for the purposes of this study is the increasing percentage of Californians who are 65 or over. To be sure, this age group in the United States at large has grown from three million people at the turn of the century to about twenty million in 1969, or from about 4 per cent of the total population to nearly 10 per cent.[3] California's population, however, was aging much faster during most of this time. In the 1920's and 1930's, for example, the number of persons who were 65 or over increased from 200,300 to 555,250, a percentage of increase of 177.2 as compared with a national percentage of increase of 82.8. During this period California contained roughly 20 per cent more aged people than the United States as a whole, and thus became one of the "oldest" states in the nation.[4] These percentage imbalances were even larger in the state's cities as compared to cities over the nation, and particularly in the cities of southern California. During the 1920's and 1930's the number of aged Los Angeles residents ranged from 20 to nearly 40 per cent above the national averages. Other southern California cities, such as Long Beach, Monrovia, Pasadena, Pomona, Redlands, Riverside, Santa Ana, Santa Monica, South Pasadena, and Whittier, frequently contained percentages of old people up to twice as high as the national averages.[5]

After 1940 this age disparity between California and the nation began to decrease, until by 1960 the state was slightly below the national average in persons who were 65 or over.[6] It is not surprising, therefore, that the 1920's and particularly the 1930's were the crucial decades in the shaping of the old-age political movement. In fact, California has been the setting for protest movements of all kinds since the 1920's, owing largely, no doubt, to the rapid growth of its population.

It is a fact of great significance that most Californians are not natives. Although no reflection on the potency of the native sons is intended, sober demographers have estimated that during the 1920's and 1930's at least, in-migration rather than natural reproduction accounted for up to 90 per cent of the state's population increase.[7] Most of the migrants after the turn of the century came from the Middle West and Plains states, and by 1940 they included millions of "Okies" and other displaced persons who fled to California during the Depression.[8]

Psychologically at least, many of these migrants tended to remain displaced persons. Although they came of their own volition, lured by economic opportunity and a congenial climate, many of them experienced great difficulty in breaking their emotional ties with their former homes, and even in prosperous times constituted a somewhat unstable and discontented element in the population. Perhaps an indication of this dissatisfaction with their new homes and strong emotional attachment to their old ones is the appearance of those unique phenomena on the California scene, the state societies. These societies, which began to appear in the 1880's, are large, loosely organized bodies of people who have little in common except the accident of having lived in the same state before moving to California. The annual meetings or picnics of these state societies have attracted huge turnouts, obviously reflecting the great satisfaction members derived from mingling once more with fellow Iowans, Nebraskans, or Dakotans, regardless of whether or not they had ever before laid eyes on the particular persons they chanced to meet at such affairs.[9] Merely meeting and mingling with "their own kind" once again seemed to do much to fill the psychological void created by breaking home ties.

For several reasons elderly migrants suffered most acutely from feelings of uprootedness and were the most enthusiastic members of the state societies. The old people had usually lived longer in their home states and had put down deeper roots there. In most cases their children were already grown and were not with them to help cushion the shock of adjusting to new surroundings and to aid in the cultivation of new acquaintances. Furthermore, the social structures of most rapidly growing California communities, especially those in southern California, were fluid and chaotic, and hence gave aged newcomers little help in orienting themselves. Finally, the elderly often did not have a regular occupation to take up their time and ease their loneliness. In many cases, they came to California not to work but to retire. But the anticipated pleasures of retirement often proved illusory. It is no wonder, then, that the various state society picnics often seemed to be primarily aggregations of aimless elders with time on their hands. In fact, a direct outgrowth of the state societies was the enormously popular Old Folks Picnic Association founded in the 1920's by C. H. Parsons for the specific purpose of dealing with the social and psychological problems of California's elderly citizens.[10]

That the older age groups in the nation and state have great problems there can be no doubt. The physical effects of growing old have always been difficult crosses to bear, and modern society with its extreme positive emphasis on youthfulness, activity, and beauty has exacerbated the problems of enduring what some gerontologists have described as the "insults" of age.[11] Ironically, whereas modern society, with its scientific and medical proficiency, has maximized a person's life span, it seems to have minimized his chances of enjoying his old age. Strenuously as the older generations in times past labored to bring modern urban-industrial society to birth, their rewards have been small. Instead of rewards the new society has visited on them a series of deprivations and a number of revolutionary changes in their basic way of life.

First came changes in family life. The new urban family is far less cohesive than the old rural or small town family, and the aged person plays an insignificant role in it.[12] Indeed, as soon as he retires he becomes a burden to his children, and the mutual realization of this fact tends to bring about a widespread attenuation of family ties and a loss of emotional security and affection at a time in the aged person's life when such psychological needs are very great.[13] That relations between parents and children often become strained over the issue of economic support of the older generation does much to explain the rising popularity of public old-age assistance programs, although such programs probably do little to reestablish kinship bonds between the generations.[14]

Second, the aged person has suffered great changes in his community life. Reared in a semiagrarian society that honored its elders, he has matured in an urban-industrial society that honors mainly a person's achievements and financial success. Since most of today's old people are relatively inactive and often poor, they have undergone a sharp loss of status and have been denied important social roles.[15] In short, they are no longer deemed wise, but old-fashioned; their life experiences seem of little use in solving the problems of a new society, and the leadership positions go instead to members of the younger generation. Denied meaningful participation in community life, and often segregated into a special housing district or retirement colony, the aged person tends either to drift into an emotional limbo of his own making or to join others like him in old-age social organizations or political protest movements.[16]

Third, and perhaps most important, the aged person has suffered great changes in his work life. Industrial organizations have been notoriously reluctant to employ older workers,[17] and since work in the American ethos is the touchstone of respectability, it is not surprising that millions of aging employees have strenuously resisted forced retirement and the loss of status that inevitably ensues. Retirement, furthermore, means the loss of a significant social role and of the feeling of usefulness meaningful role-playing brings. It also destroys the retired person's pattern of life activity by removing its vital center, the job, and engulfs him in endless hours of leisure from which he is unprepared to benefit. It deprives the retiree of his sense of social identity, since society tends to categorize the individual by the work he does. And it disrupts his life-long pattern of association, since the majority of one's associates are typically those with whom one works.[18] Finally, if social deprivations such as these make unemployment extremely unpleasant for the older age groups, it becomes nearly intolerable when accompanied by economic hardship.

The progressive impoverishment of America's aged in the present century is easily documented. In 1922 it was estimated that one-third of the persons aged 65 or over in the nation were dependent wholly or in part on others for their livelihood.[19] By 1930 the proportion had grown to two-fifths, by 1935 to one-half, and by 1940 to over two-thirds.[20] After 1940 the situation was eased somewhat by the development of old-age security programs, but by the mid-1960's the income level of this group was still dismally low.[21] The causes of this impoverishment are easily discerned. Before the inauguration of Social Security, the unemployed old person had three possible sources of economic security—his own savings, family support, or an industrial pension. Up to 1940 at least, all three proved grossly inadequate, the first and second because wages were generally low compared to living costs, and the third because industrial pensions failed to cover the vast majority of workers.[22]

The psychological strains created by poverty among the aged were very great. The necessity of depending on relatives for support—and about one-half of the dependent aged in the 1920's and 1930's were in this category—created severe tensions within families, especially since the generally low wage levels made it difficult for a family head to support his children adequately, to say nothing of his aged parents.[23] Furthermore, in an age of laissez faire, poverty was widely regarded as a sign of moral weakness, a view that undoubtedly brought psychological distress to masses of aged unfortunates.[24] Finally, the prospect of spending one's declining years in one of the many poorhouses that still dotted the American landscape in the 1920's and 1930's produced in many a feeling of desperation, even terror, that is difficult to recapture in this day of comparatively widespread public welfare programs.[25]

Finally, to this catalog of disasters must be added the acute problems of failing physical and mental health. Of course, poor health is a natural factor in the aging process, but inadequate medical services are an unnatural social factor that has victimized millions of aged Americans in the twentieth century.[26] Obviously this problem is related to the economic deprivation of the aged. Not only does failing health lead to unemployment, but unemployment makes an old person financially unable to secure adequate medical care. Thus he remains permanently unemployed, permanently unemployable, and permanently sick.

Likewise, the aging person's fear of losing his job, the shattering of morale that often accompanies his sudden and forced retirement, and the feelings of frustration and uselessness caused by society's refusal to allow a retired person to participate meaningfully in community affairs all combine with his failing physical faculties to undermine his mental health.[27] Most gerontologists have consistently asserted that if the aged were allowed to participate actively in public affairs, especially by serving in advisory roles that put their experience and wisdom to use, both society in general and the older age groups in particular would benefit appreciably.[28] Nevertheless, modern society has largely refused to allow the aged to participate. When confronted with such psychological and social disabilities, the aged person has only two real options open to him: to withdraw into an emotional limbo of apathy and infantilism, or to seek to alleviate his plight by political means.[29]

If the social and economic plight of the aged was characteristic of the country as a whole, it was probably most severe in California. As we have seen, during the 1920's and 1930's California contained a much larger percentage of old people than the nation at large, and in all likelihood the social deprivations accompanying this increase were more acute in California. Family ties were probably more attenuated there, simply because many aged Californians, being migrants to the state, were at a greater physical distance from their children.[30] The aged Californian probably found it more difficult than the aged person elsewhere to participate in community affairs, since the social life of most rapidly growing California communities was extremely amorphous and chaotic, and since rapid growth generated widespread public problems whose solution seemed to require the leadership of a vigorous and dynamic younger generation.

Furthermore, for a variety of reasons the problem of unemployment among the aged was more serious in California than else-where.[31] This disparity was noticeable in the 1920's and increased sharply during the ensuing decade. From 1930 to 1940, for example, the number of persons in the United States in the 65-and-over age group increased by 24 per cent, but the number in this age group who were employed decreased by 22 per cent. In California the number in this age group increased by 25 per cent, but the number employed decreased by 38 per cent. By 1940 about 58 per cent of the aged persons in the nation and about 69 per cent of those in California were unemployed. Similarly, unemployment was a greater problem for the 45–64 age group in California than in the nation at large, with the probable result that in California the middle-aged group had a greater sense of identity with the older age groups and a greater tendency to support their political programs.[32]

Given this pattern of widespread unemployment, it is not surprising that the aged and aging in California were chonic sufferers of economic and social deprivations. As Chapter 2 shows, there were thousands of aged destitutes both within and without the state's poorhouses in the 1920's; after 1930, of course, the ranks of these aged indigents were swelled many times over by the shattering impact of the Great Depression. Needless to say, economic deprivation took its toll in terms of failing health and inadequate medical care.[33] Finally, declining physical health among the aged, when combined with the various forms of social deprivation in California, brought the usual problems of failing mental health and possibly intensified them there.[34]

In these circumstances is is hardly surprising that the older age groups in California turned to politics, or that in the nation at large they became a cohesive political interest group, even though old people in other countries have not generally been politically unified or active.[35] The fact is that by the 1930's the nation's aged had become in a sense a minority group,[36] suffering from anomie and status anxiety, and eager to gain redress from a seemingly insensitive or hostile society by engaging in pressure politics.[37] It is even less surprising that the older age groups in California engaged in interest-group politics, since their problems were particularly acute and since this particular style of political activity had become notoriously typical there.[38] In addition, the fact that many of California's aged were migrants and ex-Midwesterners tended to increase their propensity toward political activism. As migrants they were subject to being charged with having come to California just to get a pension.[39] And as former Midwesterners they brought with them some traces of the old populism: a belief in governmental activism, in economic panaceas, and in the malignancy of the interests opposing them, and a revivalistic style of political thought and action.[40]

The background of most of California's old people, then, probably increased their tendency to follow unorthodox leaders and to engage en masse in such crackpot crusades as the Townsend and Ham and Eggs movements.[41] It must be remembered, however, that interest-group politics generally produces involvement within the mainstream of political life rather than outside it, and that the general thrust of old-age politics in California was in the direction of establishing alliances with other groups within the political arena and gaining political respectability.[42] Although these tactics were less colorful than the medicine-show antics of Townsend and his cohorts, they were far more effective, for they must be credited with almost all of the political gains won by the aged in California.

If it is understandable that the older age groups in California went into politics, their specific political objectives were not as self-evident as one might expect. Because their political demands were usually stated in economic terms, mainly in the form of requests for higher pensions, it is commonly assumed that their objectives were purely economic in nature. In my opinion, however, the old people of California considered their social plight at least as pressing, if not more so, than their economic one. For one thing, the rhetoric they used in making their demands suggests that higher pensions were considered as much a means to an end as an end in themselves. For another, what is known as status anxiety is one of the most easily discernible characteristics of their collective political behavior.[43] Thus it seems that the ultimate end of the older age groups was to elevate their social position by gaining a measure of economic independence.

But at this point the California older age groups encountered a painful dilemma, for in the prevailing ethos of the 1920's and 1930's their economic and social objectives were basically incompatible. In the ideological matrix of laissez-faire, one might live on the bounty of the state, but one forfeited one's respectability in the process. If one sought to raise one's income by requesting state aid, one lowered one's status by accepting it. The more successful the California aged were in securing larger pensions from the state treasury, the more they tended to be identified as paupers and "spongers" in the public mind. As a result their social status did not rise with their incomes, but tended to fall.

If this situation seems hopeless in retrospect, however, it did not seem hopeless to the pension leaders of the time. In general their objective was to secure, retain, and enlarge a state old-age pension system while at the same time avoiding the objectionable social consequences of such a system. Basically, this meant convincing the public that state old-age pensions were not merely given to the recipients but earned by them. The theory was that the aged person had benefited society by working hard, paying taxes, and rearing children, and that society paid its debt to him with an old-age pension. It was crucial to the recipient's self-esteem that the stipend be specifically designated a pension rather than assistance, aid, or relief, for a pension is supposedly earned, whereas the others are given.[44] Although this seemingly picayunish point was granted in many states, the best that the aged in California could do was to have the system called Old-Age Security (OAS), and even that name was strenuously resisted.*

Another goal was to make the pension payable as a matter of right rather than on the basis of need. Under the second system a person who needed a pension was classified a pauper, and the state could, and frequently did, require him to sign a pauper's oath whereby he officially accepted this badge of moral inferiority. Furthermore, so long as the pension was granted on the basis of need, the state was entitled, indeed obligated, to conduct a detailed

---

* Florence Parker, "Experience under State Old-Age Pension Acts in 1933," *Monthly Labor Review*, XXXIX (1934), 255; Olive Henderson, "One Year's Experience with Pensions in California," in American Association for Old-Age Security, *Old-Age Security Progress* (New York, 1931), p. 50; Floyd A. Bond et al., *Our Needy Aged: A California Study of a National Problem* (New York, 1954), p. 330. For the sake of convenience, assistance of this type is referred to as pensions in this book. Although California still uses the official name Old-Age Security, the general public and newspapers seem largely to have accepted the word pension. This seems not, however, to have rendered the pensions automatically respectable, as old-age leaders had hoped.

investigation to determine whether the applicant's need was great enough to warrant the pension. These tests inevitably subjected the applicants to many indignities they worked diligently to abolish. The pensioners complained particularly of "prying" social workers, who were usually many years younger than the applicants and frequently women, and who allegedly entangled them in reams of "red tape," asked personal questions, and generally "humiliated" the pensioners by their haughty attitudes.[45] "Today we must bow to some strapping young squirt / Or conceited authority wrapped in a skirt," wrote one disgruntled scribbler in an old-age protest publication.[46]

Another problem was that an applicant who owned his home or any other form of real property was required to accept a state lien or other encumbrance on it, thereby enabling the state to recover some of the cost of the pension when the pensioner's estate was divided. Although this practice seemed perfectly proper to a business-oriented society, it had the effect of clouding the pensioner's title to his property, undermining his status as an independent home owner, and depriving him of the satisfaction of bequeathing his estate to his progeny.[47]

Finally, the state refused to grant the pension if the applicant had legally responsible relatives able to care for him. This provision entailed an additional examination into the relatives' finances, and by forcing the relatives either to support the applicant or to show cause of their failure to do so, it tended to heighten the tensions that already existed between the indigent aged and their children.[48] All of these features of the California law provided grist for the mill of the pension lobby, and as long as the law retained them, old-age political activism could be described as a "normal" form of political behavior.

Or could it? As is probably apparent, all of the foregoing efforts to explain the phenomenon of old-age politics are based on certain hypotheses about the psychological and physiological nature of the aging process. The major hypothesis used here, as any gerontologist will recognize, is the activity theory of aging.[49] Basically this theory asserts that the aged person needs to engage in a fairly high level of activity in order to prevent bodily and mental deterioration. When the opportunity for activity is limited, as it is in modern American society by forced retirement and the denial of

community roles, an aged person naturally turns to political activity, not only for the purpose of reaching his social and economic
objectives but because political activity as such has definite therapeutic value. If social deprivations remain acute the aged person
feels alienated from society and becomes hostile toward it, a state
of mind that heightens his propensity for political activism. Thus
old-age politics, like interest-group politics of all kinds, becomes
self-perpetuating and institutionalized. In other words, old-age
political behavior in the United States is "normal" political behavior; aged persons are "normal" American citizens who want
the same things as the rest of us—meaningful activity, social acceptance and participation, and economic security.

Although the activity theory is obviously useful in delineating
the problems of aging in modern society and in explaining the
phenomenon of old-age politics, it leaves certain questions unan-
swered. What about the aged who are politically inactive? How
can we account for the fact that during some of the most frenzied
and belligerent old-age movements in California, there were large
numbers of aged persons suffering from all of the deprivations
peculiar to their class who remained apparently apathetic and un-
responsive to the political appeals of their spokesmen? Behavioral
science provides a number of possible answers to this vexing question that the hapless historian may call to his aid.

It can be dealt with, for example, as a problem of individual
psychology and personality structure. Different personality types,
according to this explanation, respond in different ways to social
aggression. Both apathy and activism can thus be accounted for
in terms of personality differences.[50] This approach, however, per-
sonalizes the problem too much for the historian's taste. Carried
to its logical conclusion, it would make history itself largely irrele-
vant, unless personality types were seen as being themselves created by the historical process, in which case the argument becomes
circular and largely unrewarding.

One can also explain old-age political apathy as a product of
anomie. That is, the politically inactive old person is a victim of
feelings of estrangement and isolation from society that go beyond
mere alienation, causing him to feel defeated and impotent, or
even to lose his sense of personal identity.[51] In all probability many
aged persons do exhibit certain anomic tendencies that hamper

their political effectiveness, but on the whole the concept seems more useful in understanding aged persons with severe mental health problems than those who are merely politically inactive.

Another possibility is what might be called the female hypothesis. Since on the whole women live longer than men in the United States, there are many more women than men in the aged population.[52] And elderly women tend to suffer fewer social deprivations than men, primarily because they are less likely to undergo a severe role crisis.[53] Housewives can continue in that role while their husbands are undergoing the agonies of retirement, and even widows often enjoy some continued sense of usefulness as grandmothers helping to rear their grandchildren. In fact, throughout their lives women characteristically play "socio-emotional" or "integrative" roles, i.e., roles that contribute to a society's cohesiveness. Women can continue to play these roles in their old age, unlike men, who characteristically play "instrumental" roles during their active lives and are deprived of them during retirement. Thus women may be less dissatisfied than men in later life, and consequently less inclined toward political activism.

Finally, the political inactivity of the aged may be explained by the relatively new theory of disengagement.[54] According to this theory the aged person does not naturally seek to maintain a high status and an active role in society but tends voluntarily to disengage from society, as a natural consequence of his waning physical and mental energies. Once he has withdrawn from society, the aged person establishes a new equilibrium in relation to it. The main characteristics of this equilibrium are a greater social distance, a smaller circle of associates, less interaction with those few associates, less intensity of interaction, and a greater preoccupation with oneself. Needless to say, such persons would have few grievances against modern society, since what they wish to do is identical to what society requires of them. Thus the disengagement theory is perfectly suited to explain the phenomenon of political apathy among the aged.

The trouble with the theory, of course, is that it seems totally inconsistent with the realities of old-age political activism. If the disengagement theory was completely valid there would be no old-age politics; conversely, if the activity theory was completely valid practically all old people would be political activitists. Indeed, this is a troublesome problem for the behavioral scientist, who, like the natural scientist, seeks to reconcile contradictory phenomena and to fit all known data into one comprehensive theory.[55]

To the historian, however, the problem seems less worrisome. Entertaining a less deterministic view of man, he feels less driven than his scientific colleagues to organize his data into a rigorous and elegantly consistent conceptual framework. Instead, the historian leans toward philosophical eclecticism, places a much greater emphasis on the importance of the historical context in which human events occur, and frequently resorts to the doctrine of multiple causation when attempting to explain those events. It seems to me, for example, that all of the above hypotheses have some validity in relation to the actual behavior of California's old people in the political arena, and that even the activity and disengagement theories can be reconciled to a degree when placed in their appropriate historical contexts.

In this matter of the historical setting it should be noted that the disengagement thesis emerged from a study of old people in Kansas City, Missouri, in the middle 1950's, not in California in the 1930's. Furthermore, the sample of aged persons studied were "stable working- and middle-class families, relatively affluent, [who] had no chronic illnesses, and lived in small household units"[56]—traits that were largely lacking among the uprooted, poverty-stricken, and ailing aged population of California during the Great Depression. It seems likely, then, that in many cases California's old people felt compelled by conditions of acute deprivation to become political activists, even though they may have preferred to disengage from society if they had been able to do so. In other words, disengagement and political inactivity may be natural consequences of aging under comfortable social and economic conditions, whereas alienation and political activism may be natural consequences of aging under harsh conditions.

If this proposition is valid, it suggests that historically the older age groups in the United States have been proceeding from alienation to disengagement. Whereas in the 1920's and 1930's America's aged were alienated from and hostile toward society at large because of their economic and social situation, in more recent decades they have come to enjoy a greater degree of affluence, if not greater social acceptance, and consequently may be more inclined to withdraw voluntarily from the mainstream of society and to form a distinctive subculture of their own.[57] If the aged have achieved some degree of comfort and content, however short it may still fall of national living standards, this improvement in their lot should no doubt be credited mainly to the aged political activists and their allies over the past half century. And since the vanguard of this national movement was in California, it becomes all the more necessary to study California's experience in some detail.

2

The Origins of Old-Age Politics
1883–1933

IN 1883 CALIFORNIA took its first feeble step toward providing old-age pensions. Perhaps the step was more false than feeble, however, since the law passed in that year actually provided state funds only for institutional care for aged indigents. Although court decisions subsequently broadened the act into a "pioneer pension" law allowing a limited amount of outdoor relief, or relief to persons living at home, the state legislature brought this modern experiment to an end in 1895 when it repealed the law and returned the problem of old-age welfare entirely to the counties.[1] In 1901 the legislature formalized this policy by passing the Indigent Act, which specifically detailed each county's responsibility to provide for its needy aged.[2] For the next generation the county relief system was to be California's answer to the problems of the aged; only after time and circumstances had revealed the system's inadequacies would the state begin to seek a new answer.

The faults of the system were economic and ideological. Since the county budgets depended heavily on property taxes, popular pressures were always strong to keep expenditures low. Welfare expenditures were particularly unpopular, not only because persons on relief were commonly regarded as delinquents but because many county officials believed that it was more economical as well as more ethical to place public charges in institutions than to grant them outdoor relief. Even when it became clear that indoor relief was more costly than outdoor, many insisted that the institutional system be retained lest the counties be guilty of rewarding improvidence and penalizing thrift.[3] Consequently, the poorhouses and their inmates steadily increased in number in California, even

during the prosperous decade of the 1920's.[4] Though these institutions were usually called euphemistically county hospitals or
county homes, they were often the "human dumping grounds"
characteristic of poorhouses all over the nation,[5] and despite the
fact that aged persons in particular resisted the degrading mis-
treatment such institutions afforded, they constituted an ever-
growing percentage of the poorhouse inmates in both nation and
state.[6]

There was a self-defeating dimension to the poorhouse system,
however, that led eventually to its demise. Though institutional-
izing aged paupers satisfied the ideological urge to punish what
was regarded as improvidence and sloth, it failed to meet the
practical demands for economy in government. The inefficiency
of the state's poorhouses and a chronic shortage of space and facilities drove the counties to provide more and more outdoor
relief for able-bodied indigents, until by 1928 about 40 per cent
of county aid to the aged was of this type.[7] Needless to say, this
system, though much more popular with the recipients, was hardly
munificent. The average monthly grant to aged indigents in 1928
was less than $15, and grants varied greatly over the state, depend-
ing on the ability and inclination of individual county governments to deal realistically with the problem.[8]

Such deficiencies in the county relief system gradually propelled
California toward the adoption of a comprehensive state welfare
system for aged as well as other indigent persons. The process
began in 1903 with the creation of a State Board of Charities and
Corrections, but the twin antipathies of conservatism toward public relief and toward state centralization limited this agency's
effectiveness at the outset. The board's name, for example, seemed
to equate welfare with charity, and welfare recipients with crimi-
nals.[9] Furthermore, the board's powers over county institutions
were sharply limited to include only investigative and supervisory
rather than administrative functions, and it had no power at all
over county outdoor relief.[10]

Gradually, however, the law was strengthened and the state
welfare system improved. No doubt the progressive climate preva-
lent in California until about 1930 contributed to these advances,
particularly after the progressives learned to adapt business rhetoric to their reform programs; enlightened reform, they argued,

paid dividends to society at large and thus constituted good business for the state as a whole.[11] By 1915 the Board of Charities and Corrections had gained supervisory and coordinating powers over the counties. It ceaselessly pressured county officials to standardize their procedures, keep accurate records, and develop a modern welfare system using social case work techniques to end pauperism and assure taxpayers of a return on their money.[12] That such tactics were effective became clear in the mid-1920's when the board not only survived the attacks of the one anti-progressive governor of the period, Friend W. Richardson, but eventually induced him to enlarge its budget, broaden its functions, and allow its name to be changed to the Department of Public Welfare.[13] Two years later, in 1927, Governor C. C. Young, an avowed progressive, signed a measure changing the agency's name to the Department of Social Welfare, its present name, and broadening its authority still further.[14] By this time California was well on its way to establishing a unified and comprehensive state welfare system.

By this time the state was also moving toward the adoption of an old-age pension system. But this achievement came by a very roundabout route. After the abortive pension act of 1883 California, along with most other states, seemed to lose interest in old-age pensions until the 1930's. During the interim it was primarily voluntary organizations that spoke on behalf of the aged.[15] On the national scene the most important of these were the Fraternal Order of Eagles (FOE), Abraham Epstein's American Association for Old-Age Security (AAOAS), the American Association for Labor Legislation (AALL), and various other labor organizations.* In California the most energetic and effective was the FOE. Since its founding in 1898 this "average-man's fraternity," which drew its membership primarily from the small-business and working classes, had advocated progressive social reforms that would secure for the average man "his right to a life of dignity and

* These three organizations by no means always presented a united front. The American Federation of Labor was opposed to state old-age pensions for ideological reasons until 1929, and Epstein was personally at odds with the FOE leadership in the mid-1920's. Daniel Nelson, *Unemployment Insurance: The American Experience, 1915–1935* (Madison, Wis., 1969), pp. 67, 153–54; Roy Lubove, *The Struggle for Social Security, 1900–1935* (Cambridge, Mass., 1968), pp. 140–43.

self respect."[16] The FOE was particularly active in California. During the 1920's it had over 40,000 members there, many of whom were prominent public officials, and in 1921 California delegates to the FOE Grand Aerie convention in Newark, New Jersey, played an important role in launching a nationwide campaign for state old-age pensions.[17]

The Eagles continued to serve as a major spearhead of the old-age pension movement. They willingly invested their own money and energy in their pension campaign;[18] they gained adherents from many labor organizations, thereby broadening the mass appeal for their cause;[19] and they circulated a large volume of persuasive, largely factual literature that broke down many of the ideological objections to old-age pensions and made pensioners more respectable in the nation's eyes.[20] This literature continually reiterated the facts that masses of aged persons in the United States were living at or below the poverty line; that most of them had never had sufficient incomes to enable them to provide for their old age; that many of the indigent aged were childless and had no relatives to depend on; that other methods of relief had failed, leaving pensions as the only solution; and that pensions had social and psychological as well as economic advantages. These contentions held their own against the counter-ideology of voluntarism[21] as well as against the shriller attacks on pension proposals as "incentive[s] to improvidence and fraud," "outrageous socialism," and "communistic propaganda."[22] Finally, the FOE cooperated with the American Association for Labor Legislation to draw up a standard old-age pension bill that they sought to have introduced in every state legislature in the nation.[23] Despite strong opposition the bill was introduced in 22 legislatures and became law in six states.[24]

California just missed being one such state. After various state agencies failed to do more than study pension proposals,[25] the Eagles in California launched a statewide campaign for old-age pensions.[26] In 1923 Senator D. C. Murphy, a prominent labor politician from San Francisco and an active member of the FOE,*

* Murphy was later elected sheriff of San Francisco and ran unsuccessfully for governor in 1938, at which time he made a great issue of his pioneering and long-term support of old-age pensions. Robert E. Burke, *Olson's New Deal for California* (Berkeley, Calif., 1953), p. 14; Murphy-for-governor campaign leaflet, Bancroft Library Collection of Campaign Literature from the California Election of 1938, Univ. of Calif., Berkeley.

introduced an old-age pension bill that was specifically recommended by the California Eagles, and at the same time Assemblyman Otto Emme of Los Angeles introduced a similar measure. Although the state president of the Eagles spoke strongly in behalf of both bills, his voice this time went unheeded.[27] The legislature amended the proposal to call merely for another official investigation into the subject of old-age pensions, and the conservative Governor Richardson pocket-vetoed even this emasculated measure.[28]

The Governor's rationale for this and other vetoes was the necessity for economy in government.[29] To counter this argument the pension advocates began to assert that since it was actually less expensive to maintain the dependent aged in their own homes than to place them in the costly and inefficient poorhouses, the old-age pension system was actually an economy measure. "Even ignoring all consideration of justice and humanity," declared Senator Murphy, "an old-age pension for California may still be considered from the point of view of reducing expenditures for the state."[30] This argument, though largely valid, was somewhat tricky. Because of the peculiarities of the state revenue system, which allocated property taxes to the localities and left the state mainly dependent on corporation taxes,[31] a state old-age pension probably would have afforded some tax relief to local property owners, who financed the county poorhouses, and would have raised taxes on corporations. As a result, corporate interests opposed this as well as most other bills calling for the expansion of state services in the 1920's, whereas many legislators favored them in the interests of their constituents.[32] Thus when Murphy and a fellow Eagle, Assemblyman William Byrne of Los Angeles, sponsored old-age pension legislation in the 1925 session similar to that of the previous biennial session, it easily passed the progressive-dominated legislature.[33] Not surprisingly, however, Governor Richardson, a rigidly ideological conservative, vetoed the measure on the grounds that it "would tend to encourage wastefulness and extravagance and would be an injustice to those who practice thrift and economy." Furthermore, the Governor averred, "The law at present provides for the caring of aged persons so that this bill is unnecessary."[34]

Unrealistic as the Governor's position was, his action in this case eventually worked to the advantage of the older age groups.

The pension proposals he vetoed were patterned after the FOE–AALL standard bill, which had at least one major weakness: it allowed the counties to decide whether they would participate in the state pension program.[35] Since the proposal required the counties to pay half the costs of the pension grants, it is not surprising that most counties across the nation did not opt to participate. Thus by 1928 less than 1,000 persons in the six states having pension laws actually received pensions, a fact that prompted the Eagles and the American Association for Old-Age Security to advocate a mandatory state or national old-age pension system.[36] As things turned out, the first state to install a mandatory system was California.

The times were auspicious for such an achievement. The veto-wielding economizer, Governor Richardson, had been defeated in the election of 1926 by an avowed progressive, C. C. Young. During the next four years the new governor devoted himself to renewing the progressive movement in California, an undertaking in which he was remarkably successful.[37] That Young was genuinely interested in the problems of the aged is attested by his official investigation of employment discrimination against the aged in California industries and his efforts to control this sort of discrimination in the state civil service.[38] The California populace was probably becoming increasingly aware of the plight of the aged, especially after the FOE campaign got under way in the early 1920's and a chapter of the AAOAS began to function in San Francisco in 1928.[39] Not content to rely solely on the efforts of these organizations, however, Young himself deliberately sought to publicize the problems of the aged by launching a new official investigation into the matter. Consequently, when Assemblyman William Byrne, who was also an Eagle, introduced his pension bill in the 1927 legislature, the Administration leaders deliberately amended it to provide once more for an investigation of old-age dependency, and Governor Young signed it into law.[40]

The result of the investigation was the famed De Turbeville Report. Esther De Turbeville, who directed the investigation, was an ace researcher in the state Department of Social Welfare and had contributed importantly to the Heller Committee investigation of aged indigence in San Francisco.[41] Her appointment was an indication that the investigation would be no whitewash of dark realities and no exercise in procrastination; in this respect the final report met every expectation.[42] It revealed that some 5,000 aged persons were housed in county poorhouses, many of which were inadequate and overcrowded; that nearly 4,000 additional aged persons were receiving some form of county outdoor relief, but that payments averaged only $15 a month and were administered by unsophisticated methods; and that a large but undetermined number of aged persons were subsisting on incomes far below even the meager allotments granted to those receiving welfare.[43]

If Miss De Turbeville was forceful in depicting the problems of the aged, she was hardly radical in proposing solutions. Her report supported a pension system with means or needs qualifications and flatly opposed centralizing the administration of the system directly under the aegis of the state government.[44] Instead it favored the old FOE–AALL type of system in which counties would choose whether or not to participate in the pension program and would share the cost of the assistance granted equally with the state. The maximum amount of aid to be granted when added to the applicant's other income was not to total more than one dollar a day.[45]

To be eligible for a pension under the De Turbeville proposal a person had to be at least 70 years old; to have been a citizen of the United States for at least fifteen years prior to application; to have been a resident of the state for at least twenty years just prior to application or for forty years, the last five or more of which had been just prior to application; not to be an inmate of a public institution at the time of applying; not to have been imprisoned within the past ten years; not to have deserted his spouse or minor children within the past ten years; not to have any responsible relatives able to support him; and not to have in his possession, or in combined possession with his spouse, property exceeding $3,000 in value. Furthermore, the county could require an applicant or recipient, as a condition of granting or continuing his pension, to transfer his property to the county at or before his death, thus reimbursing the county for the aid he had received. Although this requirement later became an apple of discord, it was then regarded as an enlightened practice because it supposedly gave the pensioners a feeling of having paid their own way.[46]

Modest as these proposals were, the De Turbeville Report did serve to intensify legislative interest in old-age pensions and provide solid evidence of the need for them. Nor was the legislature remiss in acting on the report. The De Turbeville recommendations were embodied in an administration-backed old-age pension bill introduced by Assemblyman T. M. Wright of San Jose. It faced competition, however, from a more liberal measure sponsored by the FOE and again introduced by Assemblyman Byrne.[47] The Byrne bill provided for a mandatory pension system; provided that the cost of pensions be borne entirely by the state; set the state residence requirement at fifteen years, instead of twenty; and set the minimum age for eligibility at 65, instead of 70.

Not surprisingly, the result of this conflict was a compromise whereby the Byrne bill's supporters accepted the Wright proposal with certain liberalizing amendments. Thus when the Wright bill emerged from the Assembly Committee on Pensions it contained provisions for a mandatory pension system, a residence requirement of fifteen years rather than twenty, and a clause declaring that henceforth the state's official policy was to aid aged indigents in their homes rather than place them in institutions. The eligibility age was still 70, however, and the cost of the pensions was still to be split between the county and the state.[48] The amended measure passed both houses of the legislature unanimously during the second week of May 1929, and on May 28 Governor Young signed the bill into law, giving one of the pens used in the ceremony to the FOE officers present as a tribute to the Eagles' instrumental role in securing the passage of the act.[49] Thus California at last had an old-age pension law, and the first mandatory pension system in the nation.[50]

The new law was entitled "An act to provide for the protection, welfare and assistance of aged persons in need and resident in California. . . . "[51] Except for the fact that it reduced the state residence requirement from twenty to fifteen years, it contained all of the qualifications for eligibility prescribed in the De Turbeville proposal. The amount of aid was to be strictly budgeted according to need, and the total aid to each recipient plus his income from all other sources was not to exceed one dollar a day. If an applicant's property did not yield a "reasonable" income, it was arbitrarily estimated to bring in 5 per cent of its value, and the county board of supervisors could require the pensioner to transfer his property to the county. The act set up a Division of State Aid to the Aged in the Social Welfare Department and provided for similar agencies in the counties.[52] It left the processing of applications and the decision on how much aid would be granted to the counties, subject to review by the state department, and also provided penalties of fines and/or imprisonment for giving false information in order to secure assistance. The counties could not, however, refuse to participate in the program, and they had to pay one-half the cost of all pensions granted.

The law was regarded by most observers as a progressive milestone in modern care for the aged, and this opinion was reflected in a number of California newspapers.[53] With the advantage of hindsight, however, it is easy to detect a number of defects in the law that were to cause trouble later. First, it left undue discretion with the county supervisors in determining the amount of pensions. This provision not only resulted in a lack of uniformity from county to county but was an open invitation to niggardliness, since the supervisors, especially during the Great Depression, were under constant pressure to keep expenses down and local taxes low. The only real solution to this problem, a pension system centralized under and financed entirely by the state, would have been considered radical in the 1930's. Second, the system, being decentralized, was cumbersome to administer, and it provided ample grounds for pensioners to complain of "red tape" and of "prying" social workers.

Third, the act contained a number of unjustified and artificial restrictions that prevented many needy aged persons from receiving aid. The citizenship requirement, for example, operated to the disadvantage of many aged wives who had had no reason to become naturalized citizens until the passage of the Nineteenth Amendment, or who through ignorance or misinformation had failed to complete the naturalization process. The stipulation that an inmate of a public poorhouse could not apply for a pension meant that an aged inmate had little chance of leaving such an institution; thus the act's stated policy of providing outdoor rather than indoor aid was partially defeated. Fourth, the act was inadequate because its minimum age was too high. Limiting eligibility to those who were 70 or older meant not only that aid would be

denied to thousands of indigents between 65 and 70 but also that
the needs of thousands more between 45 and 65 who were judged
old by employment managers and who clearly needed assistance
as much as those over 70 would be largely ignored. "California's
new law," wrote Esther De Turbeville, "will assist those who are
now too old to work or to enjoy the benefits of any old-age insurance system, but the survey worker was impressed by the oncoming
army of those between 50 and 70 years of age who are living un-
willingly in forced idleness and who ask not for aid but for a
chance to work. Their problem is still unsolved."[54]

Finally, the act did nothing to preserve a pensioner's self-respect. Its entire spirit and approach suggested charity or relief
grudgingly given by the public rather than pensions legitimately
earned by the recipients. The clause allowing the state to take over
a pensioner's property, the thicket of restrictions around the applications for aid, the investigations into the private affairs of the
applicant and his family, the necessity of swearing under oath that
statements made in the applications were true (these were often
traditional pauper's oaths in many counties[55]), and the heavy penalties attached to making false statements all suggested that the
applicants were a class of humble beggars or suspicious characters
likely to cheat the public. The new law, in short, was a long step
in the right direction, but it needed a number of amendments and
liberalizations if it was to deal effectively with the social and economic problems of the needy aged.

Despite its inadequacies, however, the law began to function
effectively in 1930, just at the onset of the Great Depression. Some
5,600 aged Californians were drawing state pensions by the end
of the year, and nearly 8,000 by the middle of 1931.[56] The number
of pensioners was substantially greater than anticipated for two
reasons. First, the state officials, perhaps operating under the opti-
mistic assumptions of the 1920's, had grossly underestimated the
number of unknown persons who had eked out a precarious independent existence instead of applying for relief, but who now
came out of hiding to apply for pensions.[57] Second, the Great Depression struck the older age groups particularly hard. Thousands
of old people in the labor force were among the first to be disem-
ployed, and many more among the comfortably semiretired with
their assets invested in real estate ventures or deposited in savings

accounts were "wiped out" by the general deflation and bank clo-
sures that swept the state and nation. For those who could qualify
for pensions, the 1929 law was a godsend, and as a consequence
there was a fourfold increase in the number of pensioners from
1930 to 1934.[58]

Not surprisingly, then, the 1929 act was at first very popular. Its
defenders continued to point out that the law was actually an economical one, since it gave a greater return on the relief dollar, and
many impoverished old people were grateful to it for saving them
from the poorhouse.[59] "It has taken a terrible fear out of my life,"
said one old lady.[60] In all probability the law acted as a buffer
against the increasing discontent of the aged. It gave them a stake
in the California political system, whereas without the law they
might well have become highly hostile to the system.

Still, the attitudes of the older age groups toward their economic
plight and the pension system as a solution were probably more
ambivalent than clear-cut. During the Great Depression many aged
indigents were not from the working class but from the middle
class. These persons, who throughout their careers had lived by
the principles of individualism and laissez faire, were now "broken
on the economic wheel" along with millions of other unfortunates.[61] The indignity of becoming a public charge was unquestionably painful for many, but when it came to a choice of standing in a relief line or accepting a pension through the mails, most
regarded the pension as the lesser evil.

Nevertheless, most aged dependents soon became aware of the
pension law's inadequacies. The pensions were small and poorly
distributed. The average grant from 1930 to 1932 was only about
$22 a month, and it tended to be lowest where the mass need was
greatest, i.e. in counties where the proportion of pensioners was
highest.[62] This situation angered many pensioners, who saw no
reason why they should accept lower pensions simply because they
lived in a certain county, and who began to agitate for an equaliza-
tion of the state pension system. Even more galling was the fact
that thousands of impecunious elders were unable to draw pensions at all because of the elaborate restrictions on eligibility. As
a result intense pressures were brought to liberalize the eligibility
qualifications. Although many of California's aged probably
agreed with a local welfare official that the 1929 law was "the finest

piece of legislation ever enacted in the state,"[63] they probably also believed in the necessity of amending the law to make it even finer.

The process of amending the law began auspiciously in 1931, despite the deepening of the Depression and the conservative reaction that accompanied it. The main vehicle of this achievement in the 1930's was a "live wire" in the Assembly from San Francisco named William B. Hornblower. An ardent member of the FOE and later state president of that organization, Hornblower had helped steer the 1929 law through the legislature.[64] Representing a constituency acutely sensitive to the plight of the aged, having important connections with leading legislators and lobbyists throughout the state, and possessing an ebullient personality and a strident speaking voice that prompted one of his fellow Assemblymen to comment that he was "well named," Hornblower was in a strong position to exert leverage on behalf of the older age groups.[65] Indeed, he was able to obtain unanimous support in both houses for the Hornblower Act of 1931, a bill that began the long and still-continuing process of amending the 1929 law to make it more to the liking of the older age groups.[66]

First, the Hornblower Act changed the 1929 law's name to the Old-Age Security Act, a designation it still holds. Although this title has never been as satisfactory to the older age groups as a title containing the word pension would have been, it was much less insulting than the law's previous title, which contained the words welfare and assistance. Second, the Hornblower Act began the process of pruning from the law those character requirements that denied aid to persons whose morals had been considered offensive by the framers of the act. The clause that prohibited granting aid to anyone who had deserted his spouse was eliminated at this time, but only after welfare officials convinced the legislators that to repeal the clause was not to condone desertion and that in many cases desertions were mutually prearranged to provide a "respectable ground for divorce." "We affirm that in administering aid the present need of the applicant is paramount, and that character requirements may act as a clog and a hindrance to an effective piece of relief machinery," said the state supervisor of aged welfare.[67] Third, the act set up a system of agreement between the counties so that pensioners could move from one county to another without losing their pensions.

Fourth, the Hornblower Act made it easier to get a pension by liberalizing the criteria for acceptable proof of age, by speeding up the process of investigating applications, and by reducing the number of relatives who were legally responsible for an aged person's welfare to spouse, parent, and child, whereas previously brothers, sisters, grandparents, and grandchildren had been included. Fifth, it stipulated that the $3,000 property limitation would apply to real property only, thus allowing the pensioner to own personal property above that value.* Finally, and probably most important, it allowed occupants of public and private homes for the aged to apply for pensions, which they would begin to draw immediately after leaving the institution. This was a notable advance, since the law now provided the aged indigent with not only an alternative to the poorhouse but a means for escaping it. Abraham Epstein estimated that by a year later some 500 aged inmates had availed themselves of this opportunity, and he was understandably jubilant about the law's results:

Not only are administrative costs kept at a minimum, but the pension payments are only half the costs of institutional maintenance. The cost to the taxpayers is insignificant. While few persons are taking undue advantage of the law, thousands of lives have been rejuvenated and cheered. Peace has been brought unto them. Old and worn-out eyes no longer shed tears of misery in sunny California. Husbands and wives are kept together and families have been united. Age has once more been made venerable. Californians can now read the ancient commandment "Thou shalt honor thy father and thy mother" without shame and with a feeling of happy satisfaction. Is it any wonder that everyone in California rejoices over the success of the Old-Age Security Act?[68]

Yet the Old-Age Security Act still suffered from serious defects. It was excessively detailed and encumbered with restrictions that prevented the establishment of a streamlined system of aid based on need. The pension grants were not uniform and often too low, and the minimum age was too high. And the act did not even attempt to deal with such problems as medical care (outside of county hospitals), employment, occupational therapy, housing, and mental hygiene. Thus though the Hornblower Act was a step forward, it left a large amount of unfinished business in its wake.

---

* The law also prohibited an applicant from voluntarily transferring his real property to another person in order to qualify for a pension.

The unfinished business was to remain for several years. The old-age pension movement, which had advanced under its own momentum and had even expanded its functions in the first half of the Rolph administration, was overtaken and arrested by the conservative reaction in the second half.* It was the tide of events as much as the calculations of men that brought on this reaction. As the Depression deepened, its victims multiplied, especially aged ones. There was a steady increase in the number of old-age pensioners in the state—from about 11,000 in June 1932, to over 13,000 in June 1933, to nearly 18,000 in June 1934—and consequently a steady increase in the cost of pensions. Whereas the state and counties paid out nearly $2 million in pensions in fiscal 1930–31, they paid over $3 million in fiscal 1931–32, and over $4 million in fiscal 1933–34.[69] At a time when tax revenues were declining, the annual per capita cost of pensions in the state rose from 27 cents at the end of 1930 to 62 cents by late 1933. And as usual, the disparity of this cost among counties was very large, ranging from a low of 10 cents in one county to a high of $4.63 in another.[70]

These increased costs brought increased criticisms of the Old-Age Security Act and demands for more economy in its administration. Critics complained in particular about the widespread practice of calling the payments made under the act pensions. This term, they said, erased the stigma of "relief" that would otherwise discourage people from applying for aid.[71] At the annual meeting of the Commonwealth Club in San Francisco in 1933 this issue was thoroughly threshed over with even some of the act's defenders criticizing the term pension and with William F. Hagerty of the FOE strongly defending it. The term was completely justifiable, Hagerty asserted, because an aged person had rendered a service that entitled him to a reward from his state.[72] Whatever the merits of either argument, the mere fact that the quarrel took place probably humiliated many pensioners.

* James ("Sunny Jim") Rolph had defeated Governor C. C. Young in his bid for reelection in 1930. Although not necessarily an ideological reactionary, Rolph was a vacillating person of mediocre capabilities who largely succumbed to conservative forces demanding economy in fiscal affairs and retrenchment in government programs. Jackson K. Putnam, "The Influence of the Older Age Groups on California Politics, 1920–1940" (Ph.D. diss., Stanford Univ., 1964), pp. 141–52; Herbert L. Phillips, Big Wayward Girl: An Informal Political History of California (New York, 1968), chap. 10; H. Brett Melendy and Benjamin F. Gilbert, The Governors of California (Georgetown, Calif., 1965), pp. 363–78.

An even greater threat to the security of the California pensioners was posed at the same meeting when John M. Peirce, a conservative economist for the California Taxpayers' Association, questioned whether the Old-Age Security Act should not be abolished altogether. The act, he asserted, was being abused by "chiselers," and in any case it had been passed in more prosperous times. Now that there was greater need for economy, Peirce seemed to be suggesting that the state should return its responsibility for the aged to the county charities.[73]

For this suggestion he was bitterly set upon by Charles M. Wollenberg, superintendent of San Francisco's Relief Home, who declared cogently, "Not a dollar will be saved if we wipe out the old-age security law." It would cost a little more, Wollenberg argued, to enlarge the local poorhouses to receive the former pensioners. Furthermore, he charged that Peirce's proposal was nothing but a plot whereby "the burden would be transferred from the members of the California Taxpayers' Association, the public service corporations who are not carrying one-half of the burden today, to the small property owner." Finally, Wollenberg rejected the ideas that in the depths of the Depression people were able to care for their aged relatives and that the elderly should try to find employment. "What chance," he asked, "has the man not of seventy, but of fifty to re-establish himself today with thousands of boys who have left school in the last three years, who are not fitted into any sort of work and who will do anything at any price to get a job? What chance has the man over fifty?"[74] To the second question the convention in effect answered "None," for it concluded that "repeal of the Old-Age Security Act without some provision for taking care of 12,000 present beneficiaries would be a public calamity."[75] Nevertheless, the idea of cutting down on the expense of the act, if not repealing it altogether, was in the air and it would not down.

The outcome of this struggle was a curtailment of the aged welfare program. Although state welfare officials tried to meet the rising demands for economy by advocating a contributory system of social insurance,[76] the proposal came to nothing as the demand for a cutback in pension outlays increased in volume. Late in 1932 Governor Rolph's Director of Finance, Rolland Vandegrift, blandly proposed that the old-age pension budget be reduced by raising the age limit from 70 to 75. Incredible as it may seem, this was the plan advocated by the Governor in his legislative message of 1933. Rolph proposed not only that the pension age be raised but that the bulk of the financial burden of aged welfare be once again returned to the counties.[77] This proposal created a storm of protest throughout the state. "The height of cruelty," one angry old citizen called it; "a very humane idea, but I prefer ethyl gas," said another. Yet another whimsically remarked, "I fear that those of us common garden variety of citizens who 'smiled with Sunny Jim' two years ago are going to wish we laughed at him instead of with him."[78] The chairman of the Los Angeles County Board of Supervisors protested that the proposal would reduce the number of persons receiving pensions there by 65 per cent; the Northern California Federation of Civic Organizations objected that it would force the dependent aged into local poorhouses and in the end cost more than old-age pensions.[79] Actually, there was probably little chance of this idea's being enacted into law, but that it was even proposed demonstrates the strength of the pressures to cut down on government expenditures.

The legislature eventually succumbed to these pressures. In 1933 it put through a drastic cut in the Social Welfare Department's administrative budget, mainly to strike at the department's director, the histrionic and radical Rheba Crawford Splivalo. Whatever the reason for the cut, it seriously hampered the work of the Old-Age Security Division.[80] At the same time, applications for pensions were multiplying at the county level, and the logical outcome was a general decrease in pensions. Whereas the average pension was almost $22 in June 1933, it had fallen to an even $20 by July 1934; in some counties, of course, pensions were much lower.[81] Even the usually generous Los Angeles County, according to one report, was steadily reducing its pensions.[82] To make matters worse, in 1933 the legislature also passed a new and more comprehensive Indigent Act making the counties solely responsible for financing and administering relief to all classes of indigents. However noble the legislators' intent may have been in providing for all poor people, the new law served only to dim further the counties' prospects of giving adequate aid to the aged, let alone other needy groups.[83]

The legislature rejected proposals to liberalize the old-age pension system by establishing a social insurance system and repealing the property limitations on old-age pensioners.[84] However, it also defeated an astonishing bill to repeal the Old-Age Security Act and return the entire problem to the counties with a sop of $2 million to be used for aged welfare over the next two years.[85] Although this bill had little chance of passage and was never brought to a vote, it seems remarkable, considering the severity of the Depression and the widespread popularity of the act, that such a bill was proposed at all. It aroused fierce opposition from dozens of organizations and leaders, and its probable overall effect was to polarize public opinion on the issue of old-age pensions.[86]

In retrospect, it seems that 1933 was the turning point in the political history of the old-age movement in California. Until that year public opinion had seemed largely to support the contention that the needy aged were an honorable and deserving group, and the legislature had responded by unanimously passing an old-age pension law and then enthusiastically expanding its functions. Now contrary sentiments were arising. The pensioners were beginning to be viewed as "chiselers" and "special interests," and the legislature was complaining of the costliness of old-age pensions and seeking to curtail or even eliminate them.* Others were attempting to shift the cost of aged welfare back to the counties, which were already overburdened and overtaxed, and where quarrels over revenue tended to become bitter personal arguments rather than impersonal discussions of public policy. The growth of such attitudes and policies goes far to explain the rise of bitterness and disaffection among the older age groups in California. This bitterness was already helping to create the succession of radical and "crackpot" old-age pension movements that were soon to erupt on the political scene.

---

* In 1933 the head of the Sacramento County Welfare Department announced a campaign to keep "chiselers" off the rolls and said that she would demand authorization from each old-age pension applicant to inspect his bank account. Earlier, San Francisco County officials had exposed a number of pensioners who were found to have bank deposits. Sacramento *Bee*, Mar. 23, 1933.

3

EPIC: Upton Sinclair and the Aged

ONE OF California's leading enterprises has traditionally been the manufacture and export of dreams. Since the days of the Spanish conquistadores, who named the region after an exotic sixteenth-century novel,[1] it was always assumed that California was a place where anything could happen, and oftentimes it seemed that almost everything did. The rapid accumulation of riches by a lucky and highly publicized few in California, the splendor of its natural setting, its balmy climate, its enormous size, its inhabitants' love of hyperbole, and the expertise of its booster organizations have all combined to give the state a sizable superiority complex. In the twentieth century this became especially true of southern California, a region that aspired to be literally a paradise on earth and a leader in everything from music to rabbit breeding, from "short- and long-distance hauling" to "drawing-room manners."[2]

Dazzling as these prospects may have been, they did not blind all observers. To some the southern California scene appeared utterly devoid of charm, a dreary panorama of hot dog stands and other uninspired enterprises operated by people who seemed as commonplace as their businesses.[3] Many, in fact, had been driven to such endeavors by the boredom of retirement. There seemed to be an enveloping aimlessness, emptiness, and banality about southern California life that was only partly masked by the strident hucksterism of the state's promoters.

This boredom probably intensified Californians' inclinations toward fantasy. A diverse and disorganized people who had come to expect something different in life were quick to seize upon anything or anybody that offered something new. In such an atmosphere, as Robert Cleland declares, "The quack, the charlatan, the prophet of a new cult, the advocate of a new school of healing, the spokesman for the novel, spectacular and bizarre . . . seldom found it necessary to search the highways and hedges to obtain a following."[4] In the late 1920's and early 1930's it was the various "nutty religions" that performed this service for many bored southern Californians.[5] Closely akin to health faddists and medical quacks who battened on the gullibility of the region's large aged and invalid population, these pseudo-religious cults proliferated like insects, and continue to do so.[6] People seemed to find in such religions an escape from the shallowness of their actual existence and a way of satisfying their need to believe that they were living in a place where everything was possible, where miracles did happen, and where social harmony, abundance, and perfection could prevail.

Strange to relate, the Great Depression did little to shatter these fantasies. Instead of inducing southern California cultists to "put away childish things" and think in terms of practical solutions to basic economic problems, the mass privations wrought by the Depression, when mixed with the emotional yearnings of the uprooted multitudes in southern California, simply bred new cults, although these were often economic and social rather than religious in character. Thus it came about that soon after the Depression broke, "Swarms of self-anointed 'saviors' poured out of every pecan grove, each with a large pink pill for the cure of every social and economic ill."[7] True to their traditions, such groups thought not in terms of dealing with immediate problems and restoring normality but of immediately solving all human problems and achieving perfection.

Among the earliest of these new cults was that of the Technocrats. This movement was imported from New York by Howard Scott, an engineer whose application of scientific jargon to the solution of economic problems soon had his thousands of followers discoursing glibly in terms of ergs and joules instead of dollars and cents. Although this acquisition of a new vocabulary undoubtedly gave satisfaction to many, it did little to alleviate the problems of the Great Depression.[8] Waiting in the wings when Technocracy began to fade was the passionate Utopian Society. Led by wellmeaning "Milquetoast Marxists," this group combined vague socialist principles (among them were the ideas of "production for use" and old-age pensions at the age of 45) with spectacular initiation rites that seemed to provide a gratifying emotional outlet for their fervent adherents.[9] Staging huge morality plays called cycles, the Utopians portrayed in graphic, if simplified, detail the problems of economic maldistribution. The movement fired its followers with zeal to right such wrongs by persuading others to join and creating a tight organization.[10] In addition, there were dozens of other organizations that advocated social perfection by cooperation, or "self-help," and still others that set up elaborate systems for bartering surplus goods, thereby doing away with what they regarded as the evil money system.[11] It was this hothouse of innovation and quackery that produced some of California's mass political movements as well as her old-age pension organizations. The first of these, which combined elements of both, was led by Upton Sinclair.

In 1933 Sinclair launched a campaign for a political program so radical that, as one observer remarked ten years later, it caused the conservative forces in California to go "into a sweat that hasn't completely dried up yet."[12] When asked by a group of disgruntled Democrats in the Los Angeles area to draw up a platform for their party that would deal with the problems of the Depression, the prolific socialist pamphleteer dashed off a twelve-point program that he declared would "end poverty in California."[13] In a masterpiece of sloganeering, Sinclair then reduced these four words to the acronym EPIC. Delighted by the program and the slogan, his listeners persuaded Sinclair to change his party registration from Socialist to Democratic and run for the California governorship on his EPIC platform in 1934. Thus was born the famous EPIC campaign, probably the bitterest, most frenzied, most vituperative, and most unethical struggle in the state's political history.

The details of this struggle and of the early EPIC movement are extraneous to the subject of old-age politics, and need not concern us here. Suffice it to say that the essence of Sinclair's plan was to make the million-odd persons on relief in California self-supporting by placing some of them on idle land to grow food and others in idle factories that would be operated at state expense. The machinery of the state was to be used to facilitate exchanges of these goods; Sinclair pointed to the success of many of the local self-help and commodity exchange groups to prove that his system of production for use would work on a statewide basis. Thus the EPIC plan was to a large extent a glorified barter scheme, a rash expedient that could perhaps justifiably be resorted to when an economic system was collapsing (as, indeed, California's seemed to be doing), but that hardly offered, as its partisans contended, a blueprint for a new, viable, and equitable economic system.[14] It contained other features, however, that appealed strongly to the victims of the Depression, generating an enthusiasm that threatened to sweep everything before it in the election of 1934.

Probably the most important of these additional features was a demand for old-age pensions. The tenth item in Sinclair's twelve-point program advocated giving pensions of $50 a month to all needy persons over 60 who had lived in California at least three years.* Although Sinclair failed to appreciate its full significance, this proposal was bound to appeal to the elderly and pensioner classes. If enacted, it would reduce the minimum age for pensions by ten years, raise the average monthly grant by nearly $30, lower the residence requirements by twelve years, and eliminate altogether the citizenship and character requirements. This and the other features of the EPIC program caused it to have great appeal to the masses of unemployed and aging Californians who were reeling under the impact of the Great Depression.

Among the less discontented elements of the population, however, the program caused shudders of alarm and fears of Bolshevism. Sinclair's earliest opposition came not from the Republicans, who did not take him seriously at first, but from fellow aspirants for the governorship within the Democratic Party. The Democrats were already seriously split between the conservatives and the moderates, led respectively by Justus Wardell and William Gibbs McAdoo, a former member of the Wilson administration and since 1932 the junior United States Senator from California. Besides Wardell, who announced his candidacy early, and Sinclair, there

---

* The other major proposals of the EPIC program were a $300 million bond issue to finance the program, the issuance of scrip money to use in the exchange of state-produced goods, sweeping shifts of the tax burden from the small-income to the large-income groups, and a modified single tax on idle land. Upton Sinclair, *I, Governor of California and How I Ended Poverty: A True Story of the Future* (Los Angeles, 1933), back cover.

were six other Democrats in the race. None of them, however, were satisfactory to the McAdoo forces, who induced George Creel, another Wilsonian transplant, to become their candidate.[15] Thus the party was broken into antagonistic factions, but however violently the regular candidates may have disagreed on many issues, they were united in their opposition to Sinclair, whom they lambasted consistently as a "crackpot" and a "Red."[16]

The Sinclair forces, united in an organization called the End Poverty League (EPL), meanwhile proceeded to capture control of the Democratic Party. Using such unorthodox techniques as selling and widely circulating Sinclair's various EPIC publications and organizing thousands of ad hoc political organizations called EPIC Clubs throughout the state, the Sinclair forces were amazingly successful in generating far-reaching and often hysterical enthusiasm for their program.[17] Sinclair himself proved an effective and tireless campaigner, as were a number of other EPIC candidates for state office. Of these, the most important for their later prominence in the old-age pension movement were state senatorial candidate Culbert L. Olson, Sinclair's campaign manager and the future governor; Ellis Patterson, Assembly candidate and future lieutenant governor; Los Angeles City Councilman Will H. Kindig, candidate for state controller, and soon to gain prominence in the Ham and Eggs movement; and Sheridan Downey, Sinclair's running mate for lieutenant governor and future United States senator.[18] Downey had long been a strenuous opponent of banking "monopolists" and a flamboyant advocate of various populistic financial panaceas. Already an outspoken champion of small farmers and other economically depressed groups, he would soon become an even noisier champion of the older age groups.[19] His greatest gift was spellbinding oratory that helped to make the platform team of "Uppie and Downey" a most effective one.

Equally effective was Sinclair's open courting of the aged. Although EPIC supposedly was not designed to appeal to any particular group at the expense of others, Sinclair made an obvious exception for the aged.[20] He seems to have been sincerely concerned about the plight of the indigent aged when he made pensions of $50 a month one of his original EPIC planks. In his tract *I, Governor of California and How I Ended Poverty* he candidly solicited "the votes of all persons in California over the age of sixty who are dependent upon their labor or upon charity for a living."[21] Furthermore, he often criticized the existing old-age pension as niggardly and the Old-Age Security Act as humiliating, although he was less than forthright in explaining how his own proposed pension plan would be an improvement over the existing law.* There was widespread public support in California for both state and national old-age pensions, and Sinclair no doubt profited greatly during the primary campaign by his wholehearted support of them.[22]

With his energetic promulgation of the EPIC program, Sinclair astounded and dismayed his opponents by easily winning the nomination. The Sinclair forces then placed themselves in control of the party and at the state convention secured the unanimous passage of a platform that "contained in abbreviated, generalized form, every essential point of the EPIC Plan."[23] It was also a platform endorsed by every major faction of the state Democratic Party except the one led by Justus Wardell.[24] But this harmony was short-lived. Soon influential Democrats deserted Sinclair in droves, castigated him as a dangerous radical, publicly repudiated his program, and in many cases openly supported the Republicans.†

---

* *EPIC News*, June 4, 1934. Sinclair hedged deftly on such questions as whether his old-age pensions were to be paid in money, scrip, or commodities; whether a person would have to retire from employment in order to draw a pension; and whether or not there would be "needs tests" to determine whether a person was eligible for a pension. *Ibid.*, June 4, July 2, July 6, Aug. 6, 1934.

† See Sinclair's *I, Candidate for Governor and How I Got Licked* (Pasadena, Calif., 1934), pp. 146–47, and Ronald E. Chinn, "The Sinclair Campaign of 1934" (M.A. thesis, Stanford Univ., 1937), pp. 93–94. The most serious of these defections was that of George Creel, who asserted that the Democratic platform was a repudiation of EPIC and that Sinclair's pamphlet "Immediate EPIC," published after the convention, constituted a betrayal of the party because it reiterated Sinclair's original program. Sinclair, *I, Candidate*, pp. 176–78; Creel, *Rebel at Large* (New York, 1947), pp. 286–88. No one else then or since has thought of the Democratic platform as a repudiation of the EPIC program. Indeed, it is difficult to believe that even Creel really believed his own allegation. The state Democratic convention was dominated by EPIC men, whose slogan was "No Compromise" and who were unlikely to abandon a program by which Sinclair had won a primary election in order to adopt the one that had caused his opponents to lose it. A less critical assessment of Creel's action is given in Clarence F. McIntosh, "Upton Sinclair and the EPIC Movement" (Ph.D. diss., Stanford Univ., 1955), pp. 204–5, 287.

The Republicans, of course, were also out to defeat Sinclair. Although several progressives had run in the primary, the Republicans had chosen as their candidate Governor Frank Merriam, purportedly a reactionary but one who refrained from vilifying his opponent. One progressive Republican candidate, Raymond Haight, had cross-filed successfully on the Commonwealth Party ticket and continued to seek the governorship in the fall election; he, too, refrained from the grosser excesses of the campaign.

Many Republicans, however, felt few such compunctions. It would be pointless to catalog all of the smears and falsehoods used against Sinclair by his political opposition and enthusiastically propagated by the press.[25] It is enough to note that after combing his voluminous writings for sentences they usually misquoted or quoted out of context, Sinclair's opponents reported to millions of voters that Sinclair was mentally defective and a physical invalid, so that the EPIC slogan should be changed to "Epileptic"; deliberately propagating an unworkable plan that would "wreck the state" and instead of ending poverty in California would "end California in poverty"; plotting to import a tatterdemalion army of proletarian hoboes into the state whose EPIC slogan would be "Easy Pickings in California"; and a Communist conspirator to whom the real meaning of EPIC was "End Property, Introduce Communism." In addition various ministers of the gospel and other "pious" folk led by a certain Martin Luther Thomas ("spouting Thomas," Sinclair called him) twisted quotations from Sinclair's books to show that he was a militant atheist and a "free lover." The near-paranoid unscrupulousness of the campaign was described by a newspaperman who reported from Los Angeles on the eve of the election:

A reign of unreason bordering on hysteria has this spreading city in its grip as the nation's ugliest campaign approaches its zero hour. The "Stop Sinclair" movement has become a phobia, lacking humor, fairness, and even a sense of reality. Here one feels himself dwelling in a beleaguered town with the enemy pounding at the gates. Convinced that this is not politics but war, the defenders excuse their excesses on the ground that in war all's fair.[26]

In addition to laboring under these handicaps, Sinclair also committed some serious blunders. He made little attempt to placate the hostile elements in his party or to appeal even to the moderate and liberal editors in the state for a better press. Instead, he seemed to place too much faith in his own platform persuasiveness, and to be misled by the near-hysterical enthusiasm he often generated at political rallies. He also deluded himself into thinking that President Roosevelt and other New Deal spokesmen would endorse his program. He even announced publicly that the President would openly support him, and when such support did not materialize, he and his supporters were greatly embarrassed.[27]

Sinclair's most serious error, however, and the one that may have cost him the election, was his mishandling of the old-age pension issue. Although he had called for an extensive system of state old-age pensions from the first days of his campaign, he had never regarded this feature of his program as indispensable, and he failed to realize how many votes hinged on it.[28] At the very time that pension sentiment was mounting in California and the state Democratic convention was incorporating a pension plank in the party platform, Sinclair, in a curious exercise in bad timing, decided to soft-pedal the entire issue.[29] His avowed reason for doing so was that during the summer President Roosevelt had promised to recommend the passage of a national social insurance law at the next session of Congress. In Sinclair's opinion, a national old-age pension law would make a state system unnecessary; thus any state action on pensions should be postponed until Congress had made its decision.[30] Although such a course apparently seemed sensible to Sinclair, it was actually a tactical error. If Congress failed to act on President Roosevelt's suggestion, the California aged, barring the calling of an extra session of the state legislature, would have to wait two additional years before Sinclair's original old-age proposal could be acted on. Not surprisingly, his enemies immediately began to castigate him for cynically abandoning the suffering elders to their plight,[31] and in this fateful decision Sinclair forfeited the initiative on this vital issue to his political opponents.

They were quick to seize it. Frank Merriam, obviously alarmed by Sinclair's primary victory and the groundswell of radical sentiment it seemed to reflect, assumed a liberal stance in which he began to endorse "everyone and every movement which might bring in a few votes."[32] Shrewdly summoning a special session of the legislature in the early fall, he submitted a program along the lines of the New Deal and secured the passage of a showy but meaningless resolution memorializing Congress to pass a national

old-age pension law.[33] Thus at the very time that Sinclair was re-
linquishing his leadership on the pension issue, Merriam was
eagerly embracing the issue and elevating it to a position of car-
dinal importance in his campaign. In so doing, he probably persuaded masses of aged voters to leave the Sinclair camp for his own.

And then there was the problem of Dr. Townsend. Only the
basic features of the famous old-age pension plan hatched in 1933
by that venerable physician need be noted here, since the plan is
discussed in detail in the next chapter. It proposed to end the
Depression by paying old-age pensions of $200 a month, to be
financed by an extremely regressive tax, to all persons in the
United States who were 60 or over and requiring them to spend
these pensions within a month of receiving them. Thus the plan
would put back into the economy by pensions the same money it
had removed from the economy by taxation. This circulation of
currency, it was assumed, would somehow vastly increase mass purchasing power, thereby ending the Depression. To some the economic fallacy of the plan was obvious, but to millions it seemed
a panacea.

The Townsend plan's almost unbelievable popularity forced
every politician to come to grips with it, including both Sinclair
and Merriam. But whereas Sinclair's response to the Townsend
plan was honest and inept, Merriam's was mendacious and shrewd.
To be sure, Sinclair at first tried to dodge the issue by asserting,
truthfully enough, that the Townsend plan was national rather
than statewide in scope, but when he was asked what he thought
of the merits of the plan, he candidly called it a "complete delu-
sion," singling out its tax provision in particular as "an abomina-
tion."[34] Later in the campaign Sinclair tried to curry favor with
the Townsendites by making it appear that he had not spoken
so unkindly of the plan,* and other EPIC men, the most important

---

* *EPIC News*, Oct. 1, Oct. 8, and Oct. 22, 1934; *The Modern Crusader*, Nov. 3,
1934. Townsend rebuffed all of Sinclair's conciliatory overtures and replied to
Sinclair's criticisms of his plan by declaring that "the Sinclair plan would bring
to California every indigent old person who could possibly make their way
here in order to participate in California's pension, . . . [whereas] self-supporting people . . . will be leaving the state, because of other features of the Sinclair
plan detrimental to business and industry." Redlands *Daily Facts*, Oct. 5, 1934.
See also Clarence F. McIntosh, "Upton Sinclair and the EPIC Movement" (Ph.D.
diss., Stanford Univ., 1955), pp. 228–31.

of whom was Sheridan Downey, openly supported it.[35] The damage had been done, however, for Sinclair was already identified as an enemy by thousands of Townsendites, who began to look elsewhere for a candidate more sympathetic to their proposals. They did not have far to look, for both Merriam and Haight unhesitatingly endorsed the plan.

Or did they? If endorsement means a stated belief in the workability of the plan, neither Haight nor Merriam could qualify, for neither seems to have made such a statement during the 1934 campaign. But if endorsement means to advocate the passage of the proposal, then Haight does qualify. "The best way to see whether it's any good," he said of the plan, "is to try it."[36] The extent of Merriam's and the Republicans' endorsement, however, was a recommendation that the plan be carefully studied by the federal government.[37] Of course, Merriam's misleading endorsement was meaningless so far as helping secure the plan's passage was concerned; if anything, it should have served to support Sinclair's original assertion that the Townsend plan was entirely a national proposal having nothing to do with the California gubernatorial race. Although it is difficult to disagree with Sinclair's condemnation of Merriam's support of the plan as "hypocrisy," the cleverness of Merriam's statement must be conceded.[38] It made no commitment to the Townsendites aside from the promise to deliver another innocuous memorial to Congress, and it brought him unstinted support in the widely circulated Townsend press.[39] On the whole it seems safe to say that Sinclair's mishandling of the pension issue, and particularly of the Townsend issue, were important factors in losing him the election.[40]

When the votes were counted Sinclair had only about 37 per cent of the total, whereas Merriam received 48 per cent and Haight 13 per cent.[41] All was not lost, however, for some EPIC candidates ran considerably better than Sinclair. Sheridan Downey, for example, polled substantially more votes for lieutenant governor than Sinclair did for governor, a striking demonstration of the power of the Townsend vote, since Downey supported the Townsend plan whereas his opponent, George Hatfield, joined Sinclair in opposing it.[42] More important, 22 EPIC candidates were elected to the Assembly and one, Culbert Olson, to the state Senate.[43] These 23 legislators, all Democrats except for Republican Assemblyman Ellis Patterson, would constitute a durable hard core of the EPIC movement and would make it possible for the movement to stay alive for several years after the election of 1934.

That the EPIC movement did not die with the election of 1934 is often overlooked by students of California politics. In fact, the movement continued to exist and to nominate or endorse candidates for state office until at least 1947, when the *EPIC News* ceased publication. Although ostensibly it remained devoted to a wide range of liberal causes, in fact it became primarily a promoter of the aged welfare movement, and it played a positive though inconspicuous role in old-age politics in California throughout the decade.

The EPIC forces in the legislature in 1935 and after did enthusiastically promote various production-for-use schemes with limited success,[44] but the shift in emphasis toward pensions came fairly soon. It was probably foreshadowed in July 1935, when Upton Sinclair made a speech that outdid the Townsend plan considerably. If the state would institute a production-for-use system, he declared, the government could pay "not only the old people $200 a month, but all the young people too."[45] Spectacular as this pronouncement was, it made no real contribution to aged welfare. Much more effective were the collective and individual efforts of various EPIC legislators in articulating the major old-age political issues in California and in working for continued improvements in the Old-Age Security Act. Although these legislative changes are discussed in detail in later chapters, they will receive brief mention here to demonstrate the activity of the EPIC forces on the old-age pension issue.

First of all, the EPIC forces made steady demands for increased pensions. Calling the Old-Age Security Act "inhuman" and "pauperizing," and a "masterpiece of miserliness," the EPIC leadership gave heavy publicity to Culbert Olson's bill to raise old-age pensions to $50 a month.[46] When the bill failed to pass, the EPIC legislators threw their support to the Hornblower bill of 1935, which made the more modest but still important improvements of raising the maximum pension from $30 to $35 a month and lowering the age limit to 65. The passage of this bill, the *EPIC News* asserted with some exaggeration, was "due mainly to the demands of the EPIC–Democratic assemblymen."[47] Likewise, when an enactment in the special session of 1936 brought still further pension increases, the EPIC party organ gave the credit to the EPIC legislators and the Eagle–Hornblower group. "Every assemblyman of the EPIC group went to bat for the measure," it declared.

If you approve of this kind of team work by your assemblyman, and wish to try, say for $50.00 next time, write us about it so we can tell them you are for them. Then give us your support in the coming elections. They need you and you need them.

And to the oldsters who get the increase, may we add modestly (for believe it or not EPIC is always modest), Good Luck and please remember that there is an organization in California organized FOR and dedicated to the doctrine of Real Cash pensions secured through abundant production for your use. And to the slogan that you will Eat Plenty in California. Join EPL and help us help you.[48]

Quite obviously the EPIC leaders were at last placing pension increases high on their political priority list.

By the next year pensions were first on the list. In a twelve-point platform of typical EPIC objectives calling for labor legislation, civil rights guarantees, and tax reform, the number-one plank declared, "First and foremost, the *EPIC News* is working for the EPIC pension plan."[49] This plan called for, among other things, an increase in maximum pensions to $50 a month.[50] Declaring "Every Pension Dollar is a Bullet in the War on Want," the *EPIC News* published pension petitions that could be cut out, circulated for signatures, and sent to state legislators.[51] When Assemblyman John Pelletier, an EPIC Democrat from Los Angeles, introduced a bill embodying this plan, the *News* applauded his action and gave continuous coverage of the bill's fortunes in the legislature.[52]

The Pelletier bill was, however, quickly superseded by the less liberal but still significant Hornblower bill of 1937. The EPIC forces in the legislature at first tried to secure the passage of the Pelletier bill, but when they saw that these efforts were hopeless they threw their support to the Hornblower bill and claimed a considerable amount of the credit for its final passage.[53] For the remainder of the decade the *News* constantly reiterated that EPIC stood for higher pensions and that the only enduring benefits received by the California aged were those sponsored or supported by EPIC legislators.[54] The wholesale courting of the older age groups by the EPIC organization on the basis of its pension record was by this time as obvious as it was unsuccessful.

The EPIC leaders did not confine their aged welfare activities to demands for increased pensions. They were steady advocates of other improvements in the state old-age pension system and very articulate in defining the most outstanding old-age issues of the day. They called for a more humane, less humiliating, and more efficient administration of aged welfare, and condemned the state pension system, with its needs tests and "prying" investigators, for its "barbarism, inhumanity, and stupidity."[55] Sometimes they made virulent, even demagogic, attacks on local administrators for their "insulting" attitudes and their reputed propensity to "throw their charity doles to applicants as they throw bones to dogs."[56] They were especially critical of the Los Angeles County administrators, charging them with cheating aged applicants of the allowances to which they were entitled and with unconscionable delays in processing applicants' claims. In 1938, moreover, EPIC headquarters set up a pension grievance committee to aid frustrated elders in securing their due.[57] Finally, the EPIC leaders called loudly for the elimination from the Old-Age Security Act of such clauses as those holding an aged person's relatives responsible for his welfare, permitting the government to take liens on pensioners' property, and requiring pensioners to sign paupers' oaths. They also claimed a considerable share of the credit when the second and third of these objectives were secured.[58] Clearly the EPIC leaders had now completely embraced the cause of the aged and were working strenuously to regain the following they had inadvertently lost in the campaign of 1934.

They even sought a reconciliation with the Townsendites. Although the election of 1934 left a legacy of bitterness between the two groups, and although Sinclair continued to castigate Townsend for his support of Governor Merriam's "reactionary" policies,[59] political expediency seemed to call for an alliance between the two organizations. In April 1935 Sinclair began to put out peace feelers. In a public telegram to John S. McGroarty, a Townsendite congressman from Los Angeles, Sinclair urged him to modify his old-age pension bill so that pensions would be financed by income and inheritance taxes rather than by a sales tax.[60] Declaring that the sales tax "reduces consuming power and makes the depression worse," Sinclair averred that if the Townsendites would agree to this change, EPIC and Townsend forces could combine and "sweep the nation." He then closed by saying, "I appreciate Dr. Townsend's sincerity and integrity."

At about the same time Sinclair also wrote an open letter to McGroarty reiterating his objections to the sales tax features of McGroarty's bill but noting that the bill made other desirable revisions in the Townsend plan; he then announced, "I now feel that most of the objections to the Townsend plan have been removed."[61] In short, Sinclair had made an about-face only thinly disguised by double-talk. Despite the fact that the McGroarty bill still contained what for Sinclair was its most objectionable feature, the "transactions tax,"* he practically endorsed it as it was in order to secure Townsend's support. The cynicism of Sinclair's offer was outweighed only by the foolishness with which it was received. Townsend publicly declared, "We don't endorse any socialistic program. The EPIC plan opposes the profit system. The Townsend plan represents an attempt to make the profit system function."[62] With this gruff rejection he refused an alliance that no doubt would have greatly increased his political power in California.

Despite this rebuff, Sinclair swallowed his pride (as well as his principles) and tried again. In October he made a grotesque proposal of $400 a month for everybody, including the aged, in an obvious attempt to outbid Townsend. His ablest statisticians and engineers, Sinclair declared, had assured him that such incomes were very possible under the EPIC plan and could be achieved twice as quickly if the Townsendites and the EPIC men joined forces.† The absurdities in this transparent appeal to belly politics were so plain that one wonders whether Sinclair made it tongue in

---

* Townsend called his method of financing his plan a "transactions tax" rather than a sales tax, even though the two were almost identical.

† EPIC News, Oct. 14, 1935. Among the many blunders in this editorial none was more obvious than Sinclair's patronizing attitude toward the very people he was trying to persuade—the elderly. In recounting the history of his organization he noted that he had first become popular among the aged by advocating a $50 pension, but that Townsend had made his appeal for $200 pensions, "and of course that pleased the old people twice as much." What they failed to realize, he continued, was that the EPIC pension was only to start at $50 a month and was to increase indefinitely when a production-for-use system

cheek. Yet it was often repeated, especially by Sherman Bainbridge, a member of the EPIC board of directors and later a prominent leader in the Ham and Eggs movement. Also at Bainbridge's request, the board decreed that all EPIC propaganda should carry the line "$200 a month, in goods and services at the average 1935 price levels, for all citizens over 60 years of age." It is on this basis," the *EPIC News* asserted, "that every EPIC can cooperate with the Townsend movement."[63] Although members of both groups cooperated to a limited extent at the local level, notably by supporting each other at political rallies,[64] nothing resembling a merger was brought about, primarily because of Townsend's continued aloofness.

By this time Sinclair was having second thoughts himself. In December 1935 he criticized the Townsend organization for harboring swarms of cynical Republicans of the Merriam variety who were willing to make promises because they had no intention of carrying them out.[65] The next month he reverted to his earlier (and accurate) criticisms of the Townsend plan and declared that it was futile to attempt a coalition with Townsend because "he thinks my leading ideas are all wrong and I think his leading ideas are all wrong."* Thus it seemed that Sinclair had been painfully humiliated in his unsuccessful attempt to woo the haughty Townsend and would not again risk being rebuffed.

Strangely enough, however, Sinclair did try again. In April 1936 he repeated his offer of alliance to Townsend with none other than Sheridan Downey cast in the role of intermediary. Downey, that straddler extraordinary, had had a foot in both the EPIC and Townsend camps since before the 1934 election. According to

---

was established. "We have to realize that old people are tired," he remarked, "and complicated ideas do not come to them quite so easily." It was probably Sinclair's misfortune that the ideas expressed in this editorial were sufficiently uncomplicated for old people to see through them with perfect clarity.

* *EPIC News*, Jan. 20, 1935. In April Sinclair also attacked the McGroarty bill, which was before Congress, but his position was ambiguous. He criticized the bill for purporting to follow the Townsend plan when it actually did not, since it provided for old-age pensions up to a maximum of $200 a month, whereas the Townsend plan set $200 as a minimum. It is difficult to tell whether Sinclair opposed the bill because it was based on the Townsend plan idea or because it was a betrayal of the plan, as Townsend himself later charged (*ibid.*, Apr. 20, 1936). The Townsend plan invariably inflicted on Sinclair the curse of ambivalence; as a result he gained the support of neither its friends nor its enemies.

two somewhat cynical observers, "As soon as he discovered that the Townsend organization was growing by leaps and bounds, Downey also leaped and bounded. He leaped and bounded from one end of the state to another, combining his private practice, his EPIC mass meetings and his speeches before monster Townsend convocations."[66] Early in 1936 he published a book entitled *Why I Believe in the Townsend Plan* in which, among other things, he called for the plan to be financed by income and corporation taxes, bond issues, and surtaxes, rather than by the "transactions tax."[67] In a preface he wrote for this book, Townsend declared that he was not "irrevocably wedded to the transactions tax as the only method of raising money to finance the Townsend Plan."[68] Sinclair joyfully seized on the statement as a basis for his long-desired EPIC-Townsend alliance. Declaring that Sheridan Downey had shown him the way, Sinclair proposed that all supporters of EPIC support the Townsend plan, to be financed by "taxes on unearned wealth" and a bond issue, for one year, at the end of which those unemployed would be provided for by an extensive, statewide production-for-use system.[69] The last barrier to a real working relationship between the two groups seemed to have been removed, and EPIC headquarters waited hopefully for Townsend's acceptance of the merger.

The acceptance never came. For reasons best known to the good doctor himself, Townsend, instead of moving to support such left-wing organizations as EPIC, made an abrupt turn to the right. Leaving Sinclair once more in the lurch, he joined forces with William Lemke, Father Coughlin, and Gerald L. K. Smith.[70] In the presidential primary on May 6, 1936, the EPIC slate, headed by Sinclair, made a miserable showing, with the Townsend vote apparently going either to regular Republicans and Democrats or to a splinter Townsend slate headed by McGroarty.[71] For Sinclair this defeat was the last straw. In a bitter editorial announcing his retirement from active leadership in the EPIC organization, he denounced Townsend for supporting conservative politicians and declared that henceforth he would "leave the doctor in the hands of the reactionaries."[72] The other EPIC leaders continued to push the Downey version of the Townsend plan, apparently still hoping to receive reciprocal support from Townsend, but even they gave up after Townsend began openly to support Lemke's candidacy.[73]

By June 1936 the EPIC leaders had turned completely against the Townsend movement, and in 1937 they even talked somewhat desultorily of taking over the "moribund" Townsend clubs.[74] By this time, however, the EPIC movement was if anything less vigorous than the declining Townsend movement; indeed, it is safe to say that the latter had contributed materially to the EPIC organization's demise.

4

The Townsend Movement
1933–42

FRANCIS E. TOWNSEND was both a typical and an extraordinary man. Like millions of his fellow Californians he was a displaced Midwesterner, and in forsaking an agrarian environment for an industrial one he shared deeply in the common experiences of his generation. Born in a log cabin in Illinois in 1867, Townsend moved with his family to western Nebraska and saw his father's business ruined in the first drought years. Subsequently Townsend became a hay dealer and ranch hand in California, a teamster in Washington, a homesteader and country schoolteacher in Kansas, a miner in Colorado, and a stove salesman in Kansas and Nebraska. At the age of 31 he enrolled in the Omaha Medical College, where he studied socialism as well as the healing arts; upon graduation, he practiced medicine in the "frontier" region of western South Dakota, where he also dabbled in real estate and politics. He served as an army volunteer in World War I when he was 50. In 1919 he moved to Long Beach, California, where he practiced medicine, engaged in real estate promotion and other ventures, and suffered near-bankruptcy in the Great Depression.[1] In his frustrated efforts to achieve financial success and his populistic tendency to blame the economic system for his failure, he was very much a child of his time, but his unflagging energy, lively intelligence, skillful oratory and writing, and intense social idealism set him considerably above his fellows. With this combination of talent and experience, it is not altogether surprising that he should suddenly step forth as a new messiah.

According to a legend still repeated by historians, the Townsend plan was born when the doctor looked out of his window one day and saw in an alley cluttered with garbage cans "three haggard, very old women, stooped with great age, bending over the barrels, clawing into the contents." Horrified and enraged at the injustice of an economic system that would foster such suffering, he bellowed loudly with "wild hatred . . . for things as they were," and when his wife admonished him that the neighbors would hear, he ringingly replied, "I want all the neighbors to hear me! I want God Almighty to hear me! I'm going to shout till the whole country hears."[2] Thus inspired with righteous indignation, he formulated his famous plan to ensure that such incidents as these should never again occur, and he did, indeed, proceed to shout until the whole country heard.

This tableau, though dramatic, is probably apocryphal. The incident of the old ladies and the garbage cans was apparently first mentioned in Richard Milne's propagandistic book, *That Man Townsend,* published in 1935. Earlier the official Townsend newspaper had published the story that Townsend had gradually evolved the plan in his mind during leisure moments spent in study and meditation or with his wife.[3] Indeed, when Townsend published his autobiography ten years after the inception of the plan, he still adhered to this earlier version and made no mention of the garbage can incident.[4]

It is doubtful, moreover, that Townsend should be called the inventor of his plan at all. In a 1931 issue of *Vanity Fair,* Bruce Barton referred to a recent jocular piece in a New York newspaper suggesting that unemployed apple sellers sell bananas instead of apples so that unemployed street cleaners could be put to work picking up banana skins, and tailors, textile manufacturers, doctors, nurses, and others could be put to work repairing damages to those who slipped on the skins, and at last "prosperity would come slipping in on a banana peel." Barton then went on to propose facetiously that the same principle be applied by retiring those 45 or over on half salary and giving their jobs to younger persons; the retirees would then perform the essential service of buying the goods the younger generation produced.[5] "Let young men do the work and old men loaf," Barton wisecracked, probably never dreaming how closely his joke would resemble Townsend's slogan, "Youth for Work and Age for Leisure.'"

At the same time, Stuart McCord copyrighted a plan calling for a national old-age pension system, to be financed by a national sales tax, as a cure for the Depression. Briefly, McCord's plan embodied all the features of the Townsend plan except the $200-a-month pension figure and the idea that spending the pensions should be made compulsory.[6] To be sure, Townsend emphatically denied that he had drawn anything from the McCord plan,[7] but he might well have borrowed essentially the same idea from any one of a number of California sources. Between 1931 and 1933, at least three letters calling for an old-age pension system to increase purchasing power and cure the Depression appeared in the Sacramento *Bee*,[8] and it is quite likely that similar letters appeared in many other newspapers in the state.

Wherever the ideas in the Townsend plan originated, Townsend himself must surely be credited with giving them the freshness and vigor to attract a national following. The process began on September 30, 1933, when a letter from Townsend appeared in the Long Beach *Press-Telegram*. In this famous letter Townsend demonstrated his ability as a propagandist by writing a simplified, succinct, and clear analysis of the "cause" of the Depression and a concrete proposal for its "cure." The cause, according to him, was overproduction, and the cure was increased consumption. He proposed to retire all persons aged 60 or over on pensions of $150 a month or more, provided they spent the money as fast as they received it. Thus the money would be kept constantly in circulation, ensuring the rapid consumption of all current production, and hence the full employment of the rest of the labor force. The cost of these pensions, which Townsend estimated at between two and three billion dollars a month, would be paid by means of a national sales tax, "the easiest tax in the world to collect." That such a program would call for a great enlargement of the government's role in the economy was no problem so far as Townsend was concerned. He frankly stated that he thought popular attitudes toward government should change; in an age of industrial maturity the people should "learn to expect and demand that the central government assume the duty of regulating business activity."

Later restatements of the proposals made in this letter reveal something of Townsend's tactics. For a variety of reasons it became necessary for him to raise his proposed pension to $200 a month, but rather than admit that he had been wrong or unsure of himself, a trait not to be expected in a prophet, he proceeded to rewrite history by suppressing the fact that he had ever advocated $150 a month and by changing the figure to $200 when he reprinted the original letter in his autobiography.[9] Likewise, when Townsend began to be persuaded of the regressive nature of the sales tax, he and his advisers gradually replaced it with the "transactions tax," which was essentially the same. When he finally recognized that the sales tax would not work under any name, the Townsend leaders again rewrote history by circulating a pamphlet containing a reprint of the original letter to the *Press-Telegram* but with "gross income tax" substituted for "sales tax."[10] All the while these historiographic tricks were being played, Townsend was strenuously assuring his followers that there had been no change in his plan.[11]

However sincerely Townsend believed in his plan, then, he was willing to use whatever verbal trickery he needed to promote it. His greatest skill lay not in the field of social and economic theory, where he was hopelessly beyond his depth, or even in the field of politics, where he was often clumsy, but in the field of propaganda. Indeed, it is probably safe to say that Townsend's success hinged on little more than rhetoric.

The Townsend rhetoric had four major characteristics. First, the plan was always billed as an economic cure-all, rather than merely a program to provide handouts for aged Americans. According to the Townsendites, the plan would provide more jobs for younger people by inducing those over 60 to retire in order to receive their pensions; it would vastly increase the consumption of goods by giving retired persons large pensions they would be required to spend, thus increasing the velocity of circulation of currency; and it would ensure full production and hence full employment through the actual "buying" of new jobs by increased spending. This last claim was the one that compelled the Townsendites to switch to a $200 pension figure. Seizing on some specious statistics, they determined that each consumer would have to spend from $2,000 to $2,500 annually to create one new job; thus an old-age pension of $2,400 per year would replace its cost in new employment.* Although the reasoning behind the Townsend plan

* Abraham Holtzman, *The Townsend Movement: A Political Study* (New York, 1963), pp. 37–38, 40. There were subsidiary reasons for Townsend's attachment to the $200 figure: the need for an enormous expansion of buying power to end

was entirely discredited by economists, Townsend adhered to the plan with bulldog tenacity, and the incessant reiterations of how the plan would fix everything in the nation's economy remained a basic feature of the movement. In California, the Townsend leaders also averred that the plan would solve the state's problems of relief burdens and labor disputes,[12] although these local appeals were usually played down because of the leaders' preoccupation with national politics.

Second, the rhetoric of the plan offered not only economic security but social and psychological security. Expert as the Townsend spokesmen were in exploiting the economic issues and "in generating honest anger at basic injustices,"[13] the social and psychological satisfactions afforded by the movement were probably of greater importance. At a time when society seemed to be telling the older generation that they were superfluous and unproductive, the Townsend leaders were asserting that it was the aged who had "built America."[14] Furthermore, by receiving and spending their pensions the old people would be "distributor custodians" of the nation's wealth, an important role that entitled them to high social status.[15] In addition, with their new-found prosperity and leisure, the old people were to participate importantly in social and cultural affairs. "Do not get the idea that the plan pushes elderly people into the corner and that their usefulness will come to an end," said an enthusiastic Townsendite. "Instead they will have time to enjoy life and gain the full advantage from recreation, political, and civil life, and have time to travel and get fresh viewpoints without keeping their noses to the grindstone."* Also,

---

the Depression, the need to satisfy the pent-up economic urges of a population that had undergone four years of curtailment, and the belief that the truly valuable traits of human character could be brought out only in prosperity and leisure. *Ibid.*, pp. 37-38. Probably the most compelling reason of all was the one carelessly admitted by Townsend—that the figure had to be high enough "so that nobody would come along and offer more. The country couldn't stand more." Quoted in Russell Owen, "Townsend Talks of His Plans and Hopes," *New York Times Magazine*, Dec. 29, 1935, p. 15. There was considerable shrewdness in this remark. As we have seen, when Sinclair sought to outdo Townsend by suggesting $400 pensions, he succeeded only in making himself appear ridiculous.

* Palo Alto *Sun*, quoted in *Modern Crusader*, Sept. 29, 1934, date of original article not given. This argument was a timely rationalization, since the plan embodied what was for many one of the most offensive features of modern life—forced retirement.

the masses of members in Townsend organizations were given a sense of direct participation in the political and social process, since they were often called upon to attend rallies, secure petition signatures, distribute literature, and even perform certain leadership functions for the organization.[16]

Third, the Townsend rhetoric was a masterly synthesis of political conservatism and radicalism.[17] Some of the features of the Townsend plan were radical enough, e.g. the large size of the proposed pensions; the supposed self-perpetuating, "revolving" nature of the pension system; the heavy emphasis on the role of government in economic activity; the idea of spending to secure recovery; the ban on saving; and the reliance on monetary panaceas, especially the emphasis on the importance of velocity of monetary circulation. Yet the plan's radicalism was not as shocking as it might have been, for the Depression had undermined many of the economic dogmas of the past. More important, many of these seemingly radical ideas were old and familiar to Townsend's fellow Midwesterners, especially to those with populistic backgrounds. Indeed, like their populist forebears, the Townsendites were largely conservative in that they sought to gain their ends within the existing political framework rather than outside it.[18] Thus they had to secure the support of as large a group as possible, and to that end had to appear respectable. Townsend refused to ally with Upton Sinclair because he thought EPIC was a socialist idea, and he was also critical of various "soak the rich" schemes because, he said, they would merely put more money at the disposal of the politicians.[19] Some of his strictures against the New Deal were also very conservative and were probably motivated in part by sincerely held beliefs as well as by his personal dislike of President Roosevelt.[20]

Townsend, furthermore, often used the typical conservative tactic of appealing to the past, specifically to the American pioneers, whose spirit was somehow interpreted as sanctioning his movement. His autobiography is replete with glowing passages extolling the stamina and fortitude of his ancestors and early contemporaries (including himself) in their tribulations on the "middle border," even though their suffering and hardships tended to make those endured by his immediate followers seem trivial by comparison.[21] Finally, several features of the Townsend plan itself were economically conservative: it was to be financed by increased taxes, not by deficit spending; it did not "soak the rich" but relied at least initially on the sales tax; it called for "annuities" rather than a "dole," thereby attempting to preserve the self-respect of its beneficiaries; and it did not propose to create any new agencies, unlike the New Deal with its burgeoning bureaucracy. All told, the conservative-radical synthesis achieved by Townsend was almost certainly of great importance in building the strength of his movement.

Fourth, the rhetoric of the plan was often religious in character and tended to elevate Townsend to godlike stature. Many of the Townsend spokesmen were Christian ministers, a fact that gave the plan a respectable and conservative appearance and made Townsend rallies resemble religious revival meetings.[22] But it was Townsend himself who took on the most obvious trappings of divinity. He had great assets that could be built up to a transcendent significance in the hands of shrewd propagandists. As a physician he could easily be made to appear as a social healer ministering to the needs of a sick society.[23] In addition, his colorful personality and his position as the leader of a nationwide movement made it easy to bill him as a great American patriot. The *National Townsend Weekly* frequently ran full-page spreads of pictures of national heroes like Washington, Jefferson, Lincoln, Theodore Roosevelt, Woodrow Wilson, Clara Barton, Frances Willard, and Susan B. Anthony, with Townsend's photograph prominently placed in the center of the page. As if the visual impact of such a display was not enough, the caption left no doubt that Townsend was at least as great as the other heroes. The attempt to associate him with Lincoln was especially strong. In one issue of the *Weekly* an advertisement for more subscribers was accompanied by pictures of Lincoln and Townsend with the caption "We Are Coming, Father Townsend, Three Hundred Thousand Strong."[24]

From this point the transformation of Townsend from a Lincoln into a Jesus was not difficult. In 1934 a Townsend spokesman declared, "There are people in California literally by the hundreds of thousands, as well as elsewhere, who firmly believe that God planted the seed of a divine thought in the soul of this humble and kindly man."[25] Two months later Townsend himself published an article entitled "Peroration" that drew an unmistakable parallel between his own work and that of Jesus:

As on the eastern shores of the Sea of Galilee, two thousand years ago, a mighty upheaval of spiritual forces began to break the bonds of humanity, which had held the race in slavery to the doctrine, might was right, that the lot of the common man was ordained by the gods to be one of servitude and degradation, may it not be that here, ten thousand miles away and two thousand years later, a movement is being born of the common people's suffering, that will have as profound an effect upon the race in its upward climb toward its star of destiny?[26]

Perhaps it was this revelation of the divine origin of the plan that inspired a bard from the Townsend ranks to write shortly afterward:

> Then let us give thanks to the Father of all,
> Who watched from His throne above,
> And chose Dr. Townsend to work out His Plan,
> And that plan a plan of love.[27]

Nine years later Townsend remarked in his autobiography, after recounting some fishing experiences of his youth, "My fishing nowadays is for men—strong, capable fellows who are willing to work hard in a cause greater than any now extant; a cause that if attained will rapidly rid the world of poverty."[28] The biblical allusion is all too obvious;[29] apparently Townsend and his propagandists had few inhibitions in their efforts to attract and hold a following.

The Townsend rhetoric did not, of course, go unchallenged. The economic untenability of the plan was quickly noted and widely publicized, and need not be dwelled on here.[30] Suffice it to say that (1) the plan would not have increased purchasing power, since it would merely have withdrawn money from circulation by taxation and then placed it back into circulation again; (2) the plan would not have greatly increased the velocity of monetary circulation, since practically all the incomes it would have affected were being spent immediately anyhow; (3) the 2 per cent transactions tax would have raised at most only about one-sixth of the amount needed to finance the $200 pensions, and if the tax were increased to 12 per cent in order to raise the requisite sum, living standards for most of the remaining population could have been reduced as much as one-third; (4) the plan would not have reduced unemployment, but probably would have increased it, since many jobs vacated by retiring elders would have been simply abolished rather than filled by younger workers; (5) the transactions tax would have ruined many businesses that operated on a profit margin of less than the amount of the tax; (6) the tax would have increased the trend toward vertical monopolization of industry as a device to avoid paying it; and (7) collecting the tax and enforcing the requirement that pensions be spent would have been difficult and enormously expensive.

These objections to the plan did not go unnoticed. Indeed, they were probably instrumental in preventing it from becoming as enormously popular as the movement's leaders claimed it to be. Despite their assertions that the plan was becoming a reflection of the "will of the people," a Gallup poll in January 1936 showed that only 3.8 per cent of the nation's voters and 13.7 per cent of those in California favored the payment of $200 monthly pensions to the aged.[31] Although one irate Townsendite denounced the poll as a "cunningly prepared deception framed by the political henchmen of the Wall Street money lords,"[32] it was probably an accurate representation of public opinion.

For that matter, 13.7 per cent was a substantial bloc of California voters. George Gallup was probably correct in surmising that the Townsendites held the balance of power between the Republican and Democratic parties in the state,[33] for none of the state's opinion leaders were prepared to dismiss them as insignificant. As a result, Townsend was handled gingerly by most of the state's politicians and given temperate treatment by its newspapers. In distinct contrast with their tigerish assaults on the much saner proposals of Upton Sinclair, the newspapers, even though they were largely opposed to the plan, were restrained in their criticism and praised Townsend's "sincerity." They also lauded his positive contributions of making America conscious of the problems of the aged and proposing solutions for them.[34] Thus the Townsend movement was regarded by many as a force to be reckoned with in California politics.

Practically speaking, it was the movement rather than the plan itself that was significant. In October 1933 Townsend followed through on his original letter to the Long Beach *Press Telegram* by circulating petitions calling for the enactment of his plan into

law. Amazed and delighted by the strongly favorable reception
these petitions received from the public, he enlisted the aid of his
former associate in the real estate business, a man named Robert
Earl Clements. Claiming he was convinced the plan would work,
and greatly impressed by its apparent popularity, Clements moved
quickly to put the movement on a business basis.[35]

Opening a branch office in Los Angeles, where the headquarters
of the movement were soon relocated, Townsend and Clements
welded a mushrooming aggregation of volunteer workers into an
efficient organization and quickly began to solicit contributions
as well as signatures. On January 24, 1934, the organization was
incorporated under California law as a nonprofit corporation
under the title Old-Age Revolving Pensions, Ltd.[36] The incorporators were Clements, Townsend, and Townsend's brother Walter,
a menial service employee easily recognized as a "dummy" whose
sole function was to meet the legal necessity of having three incorporators. Thus Townsend and Clements were assured of absolute control over the organization's activities and, perhaps more
important, over its finances.[37] With these promising beginnings,
the two leaders set out to make themselves heard all over the state
and nation.

The first device they employed to this end was the mass meeting. Capitalizing on the immediate popularity of the plan among
the aged and economically deprived, Townsend and Clements
began to hold meetings in public and private gathering places in
Los Angeles. They were greatly heartened by the enthusiasm with
which the listeners greeted speeches by Townsend and several unemployed ministers he had hired to speak for the plan. It was in
San Diego, however, rather than Los Angeles, that Townsend
made his first concerted effort to break records by attracting large
audiences. Shrewdly designating this city, which was heavily populated with old people, the "laboratory" of his "experiment," he
began speaking there in July 1934 and was soon attracting thousands of listeners to his well-staged open-air gatherings.[38] So persuasive were the doctor and his lieutenants that many local businessmen and politicians seemingly began to endorse the plan with
as much fervor as the old people, and it was reported that many of
the old people, confident they had the sympathy of the business
community, began to spend their pensions in advance by buying

on the installment plan.[39] In short, "San Diego embraced Townsendism with an enthusiasm bordering on hysteria."

There, for the first time, did it become evident that the Townsend plan
was not a cause but a religion. The old people of San Diego flocked to
the doctor's movement like pilgrims entering a holy city. So far as the
Townsend proposal was concerned, "the shape of things to come" was
manifested in the eagerness with which San Diego swallowed the doctor's
words. Clements was stunned, and the reception exceeded even Townsend's wildest dreams.[40]

Soon similar mass demonstrations occurred in many other cities
in the state, and even the nation.

If the mass meeting was Townsend's main instrument for winning widespread support, the Townsend clubs were his main instrument for retaining it. The idea of organizing the enthusiastic
Townsendites of every locality into clubs probably originated with
Clements. Whoever was responsible, the clubs proved to be a near-
perfect instrument for communicating with the general membership and generating political action at the local level. The first
club was organized on August 17, 1934, in Huntington Park, near
Los Angeles; from that point on they began to multiply at an
astonishing rate. Some 80 clubs sprang up in San Diego in the
wake of Townsend's appearances there, and soon the process began
to be repeated in towns all over the state. By November 1936 there
were Townsend clubs in every state in the union, and according
to the California leaders, some 1,200 in California alone.[41]

Essential to this rapid growth was the "incentive method" of
organizing. Under this system the district organizers, or "live
wires," and the state area managers were allowed to keep from 20
to 40 per cent of the enrolling fees (25 cents per person) of all new
members, a commission that amounted to a lucrative source of
income for the ablest promoters.[42] If this system seems corrupt, it
should be remembered that many an aged club member felt adequately compensated for his membership dues no matter who
pocketed them. Club membership provided many social satisfactions, however meager the economic and political returns, and the
leadership was quick to recognize and exploit the social aspect of
the club system.[43]

Just as important to the successful launching of the movement
as either the mass meeting or the clubs was the Townsend news-

paper. This excellent vehicle for generating mass enthusiasm and for holding the allegiance of the rank and file was started on July 7, 1934, with the appearance in Long Beach of the first issue of the *Modern Crusader*, a sixteen-page tabloid edited by C. J. McDonald.[44] McDonald soon differed with Townsend over editorial and fiscal policies; in September 1934 Townsend and Clements responded by incorporating the Prosperity Publishing Company, Ltd., an action that gave them complete control over all Townsend publications.[45] McDonald tried to continue publishing the paper on his own for a few months, but the *Crusader* was repudiated by Townsend in November. On January 21, 1935, the *Townsend National Weekly* appeared as the official organ of the movement, and both the *Crusader* and Mr. McDonald disappeared from the scene.[46] Townsend and Clements kept the *Weekly* firmly under their control, and since it soon gained a circulation of at least 300,000, it was an indispensable instrument of propaganda and a highly lucrative source of revenue.[47]

By the time the Townsend movement was fully launched it had acquired several characteristics that were to be repeated in other old-age organizations. Of these the most noticeable were deviant* or autocratic leadership, or both; questionable handling of finances; and recurrent internal dissension. In some respects these factors were connected in a cause-and-effect relationship. The movement's lack of political respectability tended to bring deviant leaders to the forefront. Strong dependence upon such leaders, who were often unscrupulous, led to autocratic control of the movement and mishandling of its finances. Dissatisfaction with these conditions and demands for reform led to internal dissension.

The deviant nature of the Townsend leaders was readily apparent. According to the ablest student of the movement, "The majority were promoters by profession: real estate operators, minis-

* A deviant leader is one who is not representative of the membership of his organization in social background and aspiration and is not considered entirely respectable in the community at large. Since the membership is highly dependent on him, however, because of his willingness to endure opprobrium from the general public, he can control and manipulate the organization for his own benefit. For a discussion of the phenomenon of deviant leadership in old-age politics see Frank Pinner et al., *Old Age and Political Behavior: A Case Study* (Berkeley, Calif., 1959), pp. 10–15.

ters and politicians. The plan was essentially a promotional venture, involving the selling of a panacea to millions of prospective customers, and their organization into clubs for financial support and political activity."[48] Because they bore no real responsibility to the rank and file, which tended to trust them blindly, these leaders were free to advocate any expedient measure without even intending to make good on their promises.[49]

If Townsend himself was more often naïve than dishonest, the same could hardly be said for his partner, Earl Clements.[50] Even less could be said for a host of lesser figures, the most notorious of whom was Edward J. Margett, a "live wire" Townsend club promoter who reportedly earned some $2,500 a month for his organizational work in the early days of the movement, while privately confessing that he was opposed on principle to $200 pensions for the aged.[51] He became a distinct liability to the movement when it was revealed that he had a shady business record in San Francisco and alleged criminal connections in the state of Washington.[52] Even Sheridan Downey, basically an honest man and by no means a dunderhead in the field of economics, was not above lending his prestige as a United States Senator to the movement and serving it in several leadership capacities in order to secure its political support.[53]

The Townsend leadership was as autocratic as it was self-seeking. The original articles of incorporation gave complete control of the organization to the incorporators, and they never relinquished it. The thousands of members who served the organization and contributed dues to it had no voice in determining its policies or in disbursing its revenues. The charter given each club was an impotent document conveying no right to participate in the affairs of the parent organization, no voting power, no stockholder status, and no voice in the disposition of the corporation's assets.[54] The clubs were completely under the authority of state area boards, which were in turn appointed and controlled by the organization's national headquarters.[55] According to one student of the movement, Old-Age Revolving Pensions, Ltd., and its successors, the Townsend National Recovery Plan, Inc., and Townsend Plan, Inc., "have been closed corporations; clubs have simply acted as service units to provide the mass base upon which the former operated. Clubs and members have no voice in the policies of the movement, except as permitted by the members of the corporation."[56] The leadership's constant attempts to depict the clubs as the essence of democracy and a revival of the town meeting[57] do not hide the essential truth of one scholar's assessment: "Leadership in the movement . . . was absolute; it was irresponsible; it was inflexible."[58]

In the first years, at least, the leadership was also well paid. For an organization that supposedly owed its existence to the poverty of its members, the Townsend movement was surprisingly successful in getting rich at their expense. The revenues of the organization came primarily from dues, contributions, and the sale of Townsend literature, buttons, and other articles. The leaders were by no means bashful about requesting financial donations, and between 1934 and 1942 their appeals brought in an average of over $500,000 a year.[59] These figures do not include the revenues taken in by the *National Townsend Weekly*, a separate corporation that, unlike Old-Age Revolving Pensions, was operated as a private venture for personal profit. Indeed, it must have been a lucrative business, for when Townsend broke with Clements and forced him out of the movement, he had to pay Clements $50,000 for his share of the *Weekly*.[60] As an added scandal, it was disclosed in 1936 that much of the *Weekly*'s profit was gained from the large number of advertisements it carried for patent medicines.[61] These commodities had special appeal to old people, especially when they were linked to Dr. Townsend's name.

These facts led many people to conclude that the leaders of the Townsend movement were merely exploiting it for personal gain. But if such an assessment seems true enough of men like Clements and Margett, it seems far less true of Townsend himself.* Apparently he believed sincerely in the efficacy of his plan, although he was not above playing fast and loose with the facts in order to attract a following. All things considered, it is probably safe to

---

* Townsend, it should be remembered, did break with Clements, although his reasons for doing so may not have been as pure as he implied to the general public. *National Townsend Weekly*, Apr. 13, 1936; Townsend, *New Horizons: An Autobiography* (Chicago, 1943), p. 153. Nevertheless, after this break he moved to put the organization on a more financially reasonable basis, and there is no evidence that he ever took money out of the organization for the purpose of enriching himself. Herbert Harris, "Dr. Townsend's Marching Soldiers," *Current History*, XLIII (1936), 455–62.

say that Townsend was financially honest but intellectually dishonest. Not surprisingly, however, many of the organization's disillusioned members considered him just as culpable as Clements and the others, and sought to reform the entire organization.

The first to rebel in California was Frank Peterson of Los Angeles. As Townsend's first publicity director, he was probably disgruntled as much by Townsend's lack of appreciation of his importance as by the financial irregularities within the movement.[62] More damaging was the defection of Glen Hudson, a dynamic leader of dissidents in the Oakland area. Echoing Peterson's allegations of financial wrongdoing, Hudson also charged that the Townsend leaders were dictators.[63] The efforts of Townsend and Margett to keep people from going over to Hudson's side met with only limited success, especially after Hudson joined forces with Peterson, in July 1935, to form an anti-Townsend organization called the National Annuity League, and after he sought to enlist the support of another group of disillusioned Townsendites in Santa Cruz.[64]

The Santa Cruz rebellion was led by a local Townsend leader named Samuel J. Daley. In September 1935 Daley repeated in greater detail Hudson's charges of financial irregularities and front-office dictatorship. His charges were given dramatic credence when, after predicting that he would be removed from his position as soon as his rebellion became known, he was fired immediately by Clements. His successor, Ralph Fulcher, demanded that the Santa Cruz Townsendites "obey the rules as they are laid down by national headquarters,"[65] thereby strengthening the impression that the front-office was domineering. Goaded into action by former Townsend editor C. J. McDonald, who called the national organization a "racket" and demanded a "Boston Tea Party" to rid the movement of its corrupt leadership, the Daley faction eventually formed another anti-Townsend organization called American Recovery Pension Clubs, which pledged to work for the Townsend plan in a more democratic and responsible fashion.[66]

The year 1936 was a fairly quiet one, even though it witnessed the defection of the largest Townsend club in existence (some 22,000 members), under the leadership of George Highley.[67] The year 1937 brought a more serious revolt, foreshadowed by an attempt by Margett to disrupt the organization and by a number of quarrels in local clubs in both the northern and southern parts of the state.[68] Then, in June, some of Townsend's ablest lieutenants in California and in Washington, D.C., defected and formed an organization called the General Welfare Federation.[69] This group was founded mainly as a reaction to Townsend's ineptitude and irresponsibility in his efforts to secure the enactment of congressional legislation, and the threat it posed was serious enough to induce Townsend to institute some reforms. The resulting "council plan" in the Townsend organization brought a semblance of flexibility and democratization, but actually did little to weaken Townsend's basic authority over the entire movement.[70]

In fact, none of the rebellions had much effect on the national movement. Each took relatively few members from the parent organization, and instead of consolidating into one opponent group, the rebels fragmented themselves into at least three separate organizations.[71] Furthermore, they had no propaganda media comparable to those used by the Townsend organization, which effectively depicted them to the masses as "soreheads" and "cranks," or as subversives who had sold out to the enemy.[72] The general disunity of the rebels served to reinforce the unity of the orthodox, thus preventing the rebels from interfering effectively with the political activities of the Townsend movement.

The Townsend movement was essentially national in scope. Its emphasis on national legislation to cure a nationwide depression and the rapid growth of the movement in every state of the union made this fact understandable. But in California its exclusive concern with national politics created a curious situation. Here was a powerful, well-organized, vociferous, statewide political organization paying almost no attention to state politics, even to traditional state old-age politics. For the first four years of its existence the Townsend organization's sole concern in California politics was to induce the legislature to send memorials to Congress requesting the passage of Townsend legislation.[73]

To be sure, the struggles over these memorials were quite strenuous. In a special legislative session in 1934 Governor Merriam shrewdly induced the legislature to memorialize Congress in favor of a national old-age pension system, a move that won him praise from the Townsendites.[74] The Townsend leaders then began a concerted effort to pressure the legislature of 1935 to pass a second memorial calling specifically for the enactment of the Townsend plan.[75] By reminding Merriam of his pro-Townsend stand during the recent election campaign,[76] they easily extracted from him a recommendation to the legislature that it send a memorial to Congress "urging a full investigation and study of this plan."[77] Although this modest recommendation could hardly qualify as a complete endorsement of the plan, it was billed as such in the Townsend newspapers. Three days later the Assembly passed a resolution following Merriam's recommendation and adjourned the first half of the session.[78]

In the interim between the two halves of the legislative session (from January 27 to March 4), the Townsend forces apparently realized that though the legislature had requested Congress to consider the Townsend scheme carefully, it had hardly given the scheme an unqualified endorsement. Hence they began to demand nothing less than a complete endorsement, and Merriam responded accommodatingly. In a statewide radio address on the eve of the reassembling of the legislature, he called Townsend's proposal "a model worthy of being used as the foundation of any federal and state legislation," and urged the legislature to memorialize Congress to "approve the basic provisions of the Townsend plan."[79]

But what were its basic provisions? The Democrats and conservative Republicans in the legislature were quick to point out that the wily governor had not specifically stated, for example, whether or not he approved of the $200 pension figure, and they refused to pass on the measure until he explained his stand more fully. But Merriam was not about to be bluffed into abandoning his support of the plan; on March 11 he sent a message to the legislature (he refused to appear in person) asking for a memorial endorsing the plan in its entirety. The Assembly, forced either to support the Governor or oppose the apparently popular plan, both undesirable alternatives, swallowed its pride and passed the resolution by a lopsided vote. Although the disgruntled legislators took some consolation in the observation made by one of their number that the resolution was a "lot of bunk anyway" because it bound no one to any specific action, the Governor had clearly won a political victory.[80]

Getting the resolution through the California Senate, however, proved more difficult. There a curious coalition led by the out-spoken liberal Culbert Olson, who was ably supported by the staunch conservative William Knowland, managed to defeat the proposal on the first roll call.[81] Olson, doubtless anxious for revenge against Townsend for his support of Merriam in the recent election, was so outspoken and effective in his condemnation of the plan that many of his fellow senators congratulated him for his courage, even though they themselves felt unable to resist the pressure to vote for the Townsend resolution.[82] Indeed, the pressure exerted by irate Townsendites from every corner of the state soon became formidable. Anti-Townsend legislators were flooded with letters and telegrams demanding that they change their votes. To make matters worse, Senator Ralph Swing, a Merriam supporter and the leader of the Townsend forces in the legislature, secured three successive postponements of the reconsideration of the resolution, thus allowing time for popular pressure to build up.[83] Before long some of the waverers began to retreat. "They're putting the heat on from every angle," said one discomfited senator, and another reported, "People called up and threatened me with everything from recall to lynching."[84] At about the same time Merriam began to claim that the resolution was not a definite commitment to the $200 pension figure; the amount of the pension was, he said, "strictly an actuarial problem" and had to be determined by Congress.* This dishonest, face-saving tactic, together with the mounting popular pressure, turned the trick. On reconsideration of the measure three senators changed their votes, and the resolution passed 21 to 19.[85]

Such was the great Townsend quarrel in California politics. Al-

---

* Sacramento *Union*, Mar. 13, 1935. It is interesting to compare the dishonest rhetoric of Townsend's supporters on this issue with the more statesmanlike utterances of his opponents. In addition to Merriam's spurious explanation of the resolution we find Ralph Swing saying, "I don't take much stock in these memorials to Congress. They don't do any good." While Swing preached this gospel of expediency, Olson declared, "I won't vote for a plan that merely puts an added burden on the already overtaxed earnings of the workingman," and Knowland asserted, "There is nothing more important for us than to refuse to mislead the people. When the price of a seat in this honorable body becomes a vote for something like this, it is too great a price for me to pay." Earlier, Senator Thomas Scollan had made a statement similar to Knowland's. *Ibid.*, Mar. 20, Mar. 13, 1935. Townsend had an unusual capacity for bringing out the best in his opponents and the worst in his supporters.

though the Townsendites may have been comforted by their triumph, a more hollow victory can scarcely be imagined. The legislators who voted for the memorial committed themselves to no further action whatsoever, and there is no evidence that the memorial had any appreciable influence on the Congress of the United States.[86] The resolution probably secured votes for a number of state politicians,[87] but as one observer noted, after its passage "Townsendism ceased to be a decisive political factor in California."[88]

This, however, is the easy conclusion of hindsight. At the time Townsend hoped to use the California memorial and similar ones from other states to force the federal Congress to enact his plan into law, and for the next few years he gave his full attention to this task. The first serious attempt to enact the plan into law was a bill introduced on January 16, 1935, by Representative John S. McGroarty of California. McGroarty (a professional poet who had once been California's official "Poet Laureate") was flexible enough to change his original proposal, which embraced the Townsend plan in all its particulars, to one providing pensions of up to $200 a month and excluding all aged persons who had incomes over that amount.[89] This was a significant revision, since under existing economic conditions it would have provided average pensions of less than $100 a month and would have excluded some from receiving pensions at all. Thus Townsend's assertion that the bill meant no basic changes in his plan sounded dubious at best.[90] A much greater blow to Townsend's aspirations was the passage in August 1935 of the Social Security Act, a law he attacked with unremitting vehemence in the 1930's, but one he was not above taking credit for later when it proved popular.[91]

Even more damaging to Townsend's cause were his misfortunes at the hands of congressional investigating committees. In his testimony before the Senate Finance Committee in 1935 he admitted that he thought saving money was "absolutely wrong on principle," that he had adopted the term transactions tax in order to avoid the more objectionable term sales tax, and that his proposed 2 per cent transactions tax could cause a treasury deficit of some $19 billion.[92] In the following year the House Select Committee Investigating Old-Age Pension Organizations made so many damaging disclosures about the movement and asked Townsend so many embarrassing questions that he walked out of the hearings and refused to testify further.[93] With an unerring instinct for the inept maneuver he sought to get back at Congress and the Roosevelt administration by teaming up with the arch-demagogues Father Coughlin and Gerald L. K. Smith to support William Lemke for the presidency in 1936.[94] In this venture Townsend was so soundly repudiated at the polls that even he was somewhat humbled.

In 1937 he destroyed forever his chances of securing the passage of a Townsend bill when he provoked a split among his own followers that led to the founding of the General Welfare Federation. The split was caused when Townsend supported a bill called the General Welfare Act, a Townsend-like scheme minus the $200 pension figure, the compulsory spending feature, and the transactions tax, but continued to assure his mass followers that this bill made no basic changes in the original Townsend plan. When asked why he continued to promise the rank and file pensions of $200 a month, he replied, "You gentlemen have all heard the old saw, haven't you, of the wisp of straw in front of the ox?" He also insisted on injecting his opposition to Roosevelt's court-packing plan into the General Welfare struggle, and he generally gave strong evidence of the assertion made by one of his erstwhile supporters, Representative Harry Sheppard of California, that "the organization was not functioning on . . . an honest basis."[95] In 1939 Townsend managed to have another bill introduced into the House and to secure 101 votes in its favor (the "101 immortals," he called them),[96] but nothing further came of the bill, and except for a minor foray into California politics, the movement was well on its way to political oblivion.

With their national political edifice tumbling into ruins about them, the Townsendites sought to rebuild their organization at the state level. Using California as the testing ground for this new tactic, they launched a new Townsend Party there in 1938.[97] Despite its state organization, however, the party was still interested mainly in national politics. Its platform dealt almost entirely with national issues, and its avowed major purpose was to elect California congressmen who were sympathetic to the Townsend plan.[98] As a result, the party fielded only a handful of candidates in races for state offices in 1938, nominated only two, and elected none.[99] In 1940 and 1942 its participation in state politics was even more meager and its fiascos more complete. In the latter year it failed to receive the minimum vote necessary to remain on the ballot. Thus the Townsend Party disappeared forever from California politics without every having elected a single candidate running on the party ticket alone to state or national office.[100]

Looking back one can easily see why the Townsend Party in California was doomed to failure.[101] Since the Townsend organization was essentially a vast pressure group, its greatest hope of success was to use the standard tactics of pressure politics. The most successful pressure groups have been those that have had close working relationships with both major political parties and have held the balance of power between them. By forming themselves into a so-called party, the Townsendites deprived themselves not only of this position but also of any advantages accruing to separate identity. Actually they never were a party in anything but name, because they deliberately avoided building up any solid base in local and state political activities.

Furthermore, they picked one of the worst possible states in which to build a strong political party, since in California parties have traditionally been weak. The major reason for this weakness, the cross-filing system, contributed heavily to the Townsend Party's debility, since major party candidates often cross-filed on the Townsend ticket, thus in effect either stealing the nominations from real Townsendites or eliminating Townsend candidates from the ticket entirely. Finally, since pension leaders wanted to ensure that major-party candidates favorable to their cause would win the primaries, they actually discouraged people from voting for the new party. Under these circumstances it is not surprising that the movement was a total failure at the polls.[102]

In conducting a political postmortem on the corpse of the Townsend Party one finds it easy to suggest what the party should have done. It should have built up a following on the state level vigorously seeking improvements in the Old-Age Security Act. The party did take the first steps in this direction in 1939, when it began to send lobbyists to Sacramento and to devote a section in the *Weekly* to California affairs.[103] Although much of their energy was wasted even at the state level in agitating for traditional Townsend objectives on the national level,[104] the Townsendites did get themselves involved in one vital state issue that might have revived their movement. This issue was whether the state should continue taking liens on the property of state old-age pensioners. Angered by what they regarded as a high-handed and humiliating practice based on the assumption that old-age assistance grants were "doles" rather than pensions, the Townsendites organized mass protests and marches on county boards in the Los Angeles and San Francisco areas that greatly increased public opposition to the liens.[105] With this issue as a springboard the Townsendites took the offensive in 1940 by launching a campaign for the passage of an amendment to the state constitution that would have made sweeping reforms in the state old-age pension system. Showing a sure grasp of the major old-age political issues in California and an ability to articulate them plainly, the sponsors declared that their measure would "remove the stigma of charity from old-age pensions, relieve pensioners from the annoyance of prying social service workers, cancel all property liens . . . and relieve sons and daughters from the burden of supporting their needy parents in addition to paying the same taxes as other citizens for the support of all the needy aged of the state."[106] Although this sweeping proposal quite understandably failed to pass, together with other Townsend proposals of 1940 it was probably instrumental in securing the passage of two other constitutional amendments that abolished the practice of taking liens on pensioners' property.[107]

The Townsendites, however, failed to follow through on these promising beginnings. The national leadership took a rather disdainful view of this foray into state politics, despite a shrewd argument by one of its backers: "Even if we should fail [to qualify the measure], it is believed that we can secure enough publicity and good will to justify the effort. We think we can enlist many to join our ranks as a result of this campaign."[108] The Townsendites did not make another serious attempt to influence state old-age policies and legislation for over two years; by this time they were overshadowed by other pension movements.[109] They had missed their opportunity to rebuild their organization on the state level, and they had entered into a political decline from which they would not recover. Eventually the movement became for all practical purposes a social club, with some distinctly apolitical overtones.[110] Perhaps such an end was fitting for an organization that was always more effective in answering social and psychological needs than political ones.

It is probably safe to say, in fact, that the entire story of the Townsend movement in California is one of wasted political opportunities. With a powerful, well-financed, broadly based organization at their command, the Townsend leaders could seemingly have been a significant force in the movement to enhance the economic and social welfare of aged Californians. But in their preoccupation with national legislation of a fantastic and unrealizable nature, they dissipated this strength and discredited themselves. Although the Townsendites probably made the state more pension-conscious, this contribution was their only important one. Indeed, most of the advances made by the older age groups in California during the 1930's owed nothing to the help of the Townsend organization.

5

Progress and Reaction:
The Merriam Administration

IF FRANK MERRIAM was a reactionary, as his enemies charged, he was no fool. Neither was he a doctrinaire. This being the case, he saw no future in standing as an uncompromising champion of conservatism in an age of reform. In his election campaign of 1934 he embraced the New Deal in all but name; in his administration, his attitude toward the New Deal might be characterized as opposition in theory but cooperation in fact.[1] No social innovator, he participated in New Deal programs only after they were inaugurated, in order to make his state eligible to receive the federal grants of money that were available. At the same time he was shrewd enough to speak publicly as though he were basically sympathetic toward the semiliberal policies the times were forcing him to adopt. If his administration was far removed from the Hiram Johnson era, it was just as far from the purblind conservatism of James Rolph. It was essentially an exercise in moderation in which the Governor sought to alleviate some of the sufferings of the underprivileged without disturbing too deeply the privileges and perquisites of those with a heavy stake in the status quo.

"What we do . . . will determine whether we can have social justice without socialism," said Governor Merriam in his inaugural address. "We must recognize the fact that unless the causes of radicalism are removed . . . we shall reap the whirlwind of our own callous . . . inadequacy." To underscore his determination to institute new policies, he declared his readiness to find new tax sources to finance them. But he added, "We must recognize, however, that new taxes must be levied on ability to pay."[2] Following through on these remarks, he submitted a budget to the legislature calling for unprecedented expenditures of more than $400 million and proposing to raise the necessary $155 million of additional revenue by levying income and amusement taxes and increasing the taxes on banks, corporations, insurance, and liquor.[3] This stole much of the thunder from his liberal opponents, who were forced mainly into a "me too" position of supporting Merriam's tax program, though they did demand that taxes be raised and that severance taxes be imposed on natural resources. The principal leader of this "soak the rich" campaign was Senator Culbert L. Olson with his coterie of EPIC liberals recently elected to the legislature.[4] Demanding reductions in the sales tax and heavier levies on banks, corporations, individual incomes, and inheritances than Merriam had proposed, plus the imposition of a severance tax on oil, the liberals were able to delay the passage of Merriam's program and to make some changes in it. In the end, however, Merriam's program was passed largely as he had requested.[5]

Two years later the Democrats gained control of the Assembly for the first time since 1893, and were thus in a position to oppose Merriam's program more strenuously. The Governor, however, again muted their opposition by submitting an even larger budget than he had two years before, thereby indicating his sympathy with expenditures in the name of humanitarianism, but he coupled his recommendations with the slogan "No New Taxes," an equally popular appeal.[6] The Democrats, unable to break the no-new-taxes barrier, did manage to eliminate the sales tax on restaurant meals, drugs, and fuel. But though this measure was a progressive step, it reduced revenues, forcing the Democrats to slash the Governor's appropriation request for relief.*

It was particularly in the entire complex and confused matter of relief that Merriam demonstrated his political virtuosity. In order to receive federal funds, California created the State Emer-

---

* Sacramento *Union*, Apr. 12, 13, 28, and 30, 1937. It should be noted that the $8 million by which the Democrats reduced Merriam's relief budget was money the Governor intended to keep as a reserve. When the Governor rejected the Democrats' demand that it be spent either on relief or on state institutions, they eliminated it from the budget entirely. The whole incident demonstrates Merriam's typical foxiness. By playing on the economy and no-new-taxes themes he made the Democrats look like spendthrifts; at the same time he appeared as a humanitarian by opposing reductions in the relief budget, even though he had not intended to spend the entire relief fund he had requested.

gency Relief Administration (SERA), an agency that paid appropriate lip service to the danger of federal "regimentation" but cooperated with the national administration in carrying out its policies and recruiting personnel.[7] But Merriam also reassured the conservative camp by striking out against relief "chiselers," and his subordinates later announced that they had waged a successful campaign to rid the rolls of such people.[8] Finally, the Merriam administration made a successful tactical retreat in allowing the diversion of a modest amount of SERA funds to so-called self-help cooperatives. This moderate concession to the idea of production for use enabled the Merriam men in the state Senate to beat down Culbert Olson's much more ambitious program in this area.[9]

The advances in aged welfare during Merriam's administration must be viewed, then, in a general context of moderate sympathy for social and economic reform. A glance at the box score shows that the older age groups in California made important gains during the Merriam administration. When Merriam became Governor in June 1934, there were less than 17,000 pension recipients under the Old-Age Security Act, but when he left at the end of December 1938 there were more than 125,000.[10] Such an expansion of the rolls naturally meant huge increases in pension expenditures. Thus whereas in the fiscal year 1934–35 the total expenditure for old-age pensions in the state was less than $5 million, in 1938–39 it was over $49 million.[11] Much of the increase, moreover, could be accounted for by larger individual pension allotments. Whereas in June 1934 the average monthly pension in California was an even $20, by December 1938 the state led all the others in the nation with an average grant of $32.43.[12] In addition to these quantitative gains there were other liberalizations of the Old-Age Security Act passed at this time, and in practically every case the prime mover was the astute assemblyman William B. Hornblower.

Hornblower's most important ally in his triumphs during the Merriam administration was the New Deal. It was the injection of federal money into California's economic bloodstream by the passage of the Social Security Act that stimulated the liberalization of the California pension system. The California legislature had already made a plea to Congress for a national old-age pension system to relieve the states and local communities of some of the burden of caring for the aged,[13] and it showed little inclination in the first days of the 1935 session to increase pensions without federal assistance. When Hornblower introduced an FOE-sponsored bill on January 9, 1935, to reduce the age limit to 65 and relax a number of other requirements for drawing pensions, it was immediately buried in committee.[14] When Congress began its hearings on President Roosevelt's social security bill on January 21,[15] however, the California legislature began to take a much livelier interest in liberalized pension proposals.

Some were even sanguine enough to believe that federal funds would enable them to raise old-age pensions to $50 a month. Culbert Olson was so hopeful on this point that he proposed amendments to this effect to two bills introduced by Senator Ralph Swing, a Merriam supporter but a supposed friend of the older age groups.[16] One of these bills, Senate Bill 942, had no chance whatever of passing. The other, Senate Bill 12, was also defeated eventually, but the controversy over Olson's amendments to it was illuminating. Swing assumed—correctly, as it turned out—that the federal government would reimburse the state to a maximum of $15 a month per pensioner. If California retained her maximum pension of $30 a month, the federal funds might give her enough extra income to enable her to reduce the age limit from 70 to 65 without levying new taxes to pay the additional pensions. Consequently, Swing strongly opposed the Olson amendments because they would simply use up the extra funds in higher pensions.[17]

Olson, for his part, thought that the federal subsidy combined with additional state funds would enable the state both to lower the pension age to 65 and to provide maximum pensions of $50 a month. Swing, who had just finished leading the fight for the passage of the Townsend memorial, now led the opposition to Olson's amendment; thus he placed himself in the curious position of asserting that the federal government could afford to pay old-age pensions of $200 a month but that California and the federal government combined could not afford to pay pensions one-fourth as large.[18]

To Olson there was no mystery in Swing's ambivalent position. He regarded it as a typical manifestation of the Merriam administration's hypocrisy and conservatism. Merriam had supported the Townsend resolution, Olson thought, because he knew it was a meaningless gesture Congress would ignore; and he opposed higher old-age pensions in California because they would necessitate increased taxes on corporate interests, Merriam's greatest source of support. Olson asserted that pension increases could be financed by the imposition of a severance tax, but that the severance tax bills already introduced would "never see the light of day" because of the influence of what he termed "private interests." These interests, he went on to say, exercised sweeping control over the legislative process in California, and he even charged that the state Senate "bow[ed] to their will."[19] Such plain speech brought Olson a partial but short-lived victory when the Senate accepted a compromise amendment offered by William Knowland that would have provided for maximum pensions of $45 a month.[20] But the bill failed in the other house, and with it died all hopes of $50 pensions for the time being.[21]

On the same day as the death of Senate Bill 12, however, the Governor signed Assembly Bill 767, a new Hornblower Act. Though less dramatic than the $50 pension bills, the new law was of great importance to the older age groups in California. It made the state eligible to receive federal funds under the impending Social Security Act, and it liberalized the state Old-Age Security Act even more than was necessary to qualify for such funds. The bill was introduced by Hornblower on January 24, withstood the passage and rejection of many amendments, none of which was of a crippling nature, and passed unanimously in both houses.[22]

In addition to empowering the governor to accept federal pension funds on behalf of the state in the event that federal funds were offered, the law brought other important gains to the older age groups.[23] The most important of these were as follows: (1) The minimum age was reduced from 70 to 65 years.* (2) The stipulation that a person had to have been a citizen for 15 years to be eligible for a pension was removed, leaving citizenship only as a requirement. (3) The residence requirement of fifteen years was changed to five of the past nine years. This change was made contingent on the reception of federal funds. (4) The state alone would pay the pensions of those who had no county residence (because they had moved about) until they had established one year's residence in a particular county. The pensioner was required, however, to secure the permission of the new county to move his residence

---

* The state was not forced to make this change in 1935, since the Social Security Act did not make 65 a mandatory minimum age until 1940.

there. (5) Proof of a petitioner's age from affidavits of his relatives was now acceptable. (6) The maximum income from all sources including pensions was raised from $30 to $35 a month. A minimum of $20 a month was established. (7) The maximum real property a pensioner could own was changed from $3,000 market value to $3,000 assessed value of the combined real property of husband and wife.* Aid given under this act was to constitute a lien on the pensioner's property, but the provision that the county could require a pensioner to transfer his property to the county was repealed. Also repealed was the provision that 5 per cent of the value of a pensioner's property not producing a reasonable income should be computed as income.

The Hornblower Act of 1935 had important effects, especially on the new pension recipients. "Oh, it's too good to be true," said one 66-year-old woman. "Now I can get a pension and be my self-respecting self again." "It's just like the beginning of a new life to me," exulted another. "Do you know I haven't had any face powder for two years?" A 67-year-old man declared that with the $35 pension he could "live like a king. I can even have tobacco every day if I count my pennies carefully."[24] Others, however, felt that economy in government was more important than providing nicotine and cosmetics for the aged, and intimated that many pensioners were simply getting a free ride at the taxpayers' expense. The law provided pensioners with "guaranteed financial security for the rest of their life," said a Sacramento County welfare official. "It's a great humanitarian measure, no doubt of that," she continued, "but what of the tremendous tax load it will place upon Sacramento County taxpayers?"[25] Others revived the old-folks-as-spongers theme by declaring that aged paupers would flock to California to receive pensions. Still others registered uneasiness over the increase in citizenship applications in the state by aged aliens who, it was alleged, were motivated solely by a desire to qualify for pensions.[26] This conservative reaction against liberalized pensions would soon provoke a counter-reaction among the older age groups. The hostility that was to come was perhaps foreshadowed

---

* This was an important change, since assessed value was usually from about one-fourth to one-half of market value. The limit was later raised to $3,500, and many county old-age pension officials came to believe that this provision was too lenient. Floyd A. Bond et al., *Our Needy Aged: A California Study of a National Problem* (New York, 1954), p. 310.

in 1935 when a new pensioner responded to a complaint about increased taxes by saying, "Well, when I had the money I paid taxes—and plenty of them. Now let the state put out a little money to help me. I certainly helped it long enough."[27]

These conflicting attitudes began to produce antagonisms as soon as the Social Security Act went into effect in California in 1936. County officials immediately began to complain of the increased costs of the old-age security program[28] and to seek ways to reduce them. The most obvious solutions were to budget the pensioners very strictly and to deduct any income they might have from their pension grants. Such tactics produced infuriated cries that the officials were trying to introduce regimentation and were prying into the pensioners' affairs. Assemblyman Hornblower soon began to echo these charges on behalf of his aged constituents. Striking an oratorical pose, Hornblower declared:

It is not up to these social workers to say to each individual how many pounds of meat, how many eggs and how many slices of butter an old man or woman shall eat. If they prefer their eggs in a glass of wine instead of with bacon, that is their business. And if they have friends that give them a little free fuel once in a while or some clothing, the value of these donations should not be deducted from the amount of their pensions.[29]

Before long Hornblower and his San Francisco colleague, Assemblyman James F. Brennan, launched an investigation into the administration of the Old-Age Security Act in the counties.[30] At public meetings of the San Francisco Board of Supervisors, which were "filled to the last seat with old people," Hornblower and Brennan charged that the administration of the program was discriminatory; they attacked the deductions and budgeting policies of the county welfare director and requested that the county pay pensioners having no other income the maximum of $35 a month rather than what the State Department of Social Welfare decided they needed.* Hornblower charged that some counties were ille-

---

* San Francisco *Chronicle*, Jan. 21, Jan. 24, 1936. This demand for the $35 maximum was obviously political window dressing. The supervisors replied correctly that they were bound by the state department's budgeting formulas, since the county could only get refunds from the state treasury on one-half of the pension allotments that were approved by the department. Although Brennan and Hornblower denied that politics had anything to do with their appearances before the Board of Supervisors, it is hard to believe them.

gally paying pensions in grocery orders instead of money and that others were granting pensioners as little as $7 a month.[31] In general, he declared, the administration of the law in the counties was "beyond speaking of in decent terms," and he warned that if abuses were not remedied the old people would turn to movements demanding $50 pensions or to the Townsend plan.[32]

This warning apparently had some effect. Despite the fact that a tax conference Merriam had convoked called for retrenchment in government activities, the Governor found it necessary to summon a special session of the legislature in 1936 to deal with some fourteen matters, among which were improvements in the Old-Age Security Act."[33] Merriam had in mind only some minor provisions clarifying transfer cases between counties, but at Hornblower's behest the legislature also liberalized the restrictions on property ownership and abolished the $20 minimum pension, thus ensuring an income of at least $35 a month for all pensioners.* Furthermore, the legislature made it possible for an inmate of an institution to apply for a pension and continue to live in the institution until he received his first pension check. A qualified pensioner could now leave the county hospital with relative ease.[34] Despite these significant liberalizations, Merriam signed the measure quickly and called the legislature's work "very satisfactory indeed." It should have been satisfactory to many pensioners, at least, for it immediately increased the average pension about $8 a month.[35]

The pension liberalizations of 1935 and 1936 brought large increases in state expenditures. The total outlay for old-age pensions in California rose from about $8.5 million in fiscal 1935–36 to over $24 million in fiscal 1936–37.[36] In asking the legislature for a record-breaking budget of $446 million in 1937, Merriam predicted that pension costs would increase to $32 million during 1937–38 and to at least $39 million during 1938–39. As it turned out, pension costs were some $17 million over his estimates for 1937–39.[37] Of course, by this time the federal government was remitting almost half of these costs to the state under the Social Security Act. Nonetheless, these increases put a heavy strain on

* It should be remembered that the Old-Age Security Act did not force counties to pay flat monthly pensions of $35 but to grant pensions that totaled $35 when added to the pensioner's other income.

the county budgets, which were largely dependent on the property tax because of Merriam's no-new-taxes policy and his defeat of the various "soak the rich" schemes. The average tax burden on real property going to old-age pensions had increased more than tenfold between 1930 and 1937. Finally, early in the latter year, Del Norte County found itself unable to meet its pension obligations. This jeopardized the payment of the entire federal old-age assistance grant to California, since the Social Security Board had ruled that pensions had to be paid uniformly throughout the state if federal assistance was to be granted.[38] Though the legislature was able to avert the crisis in the 1937 session by passing an emergency act making the state remittances to the counties for pensions payable in advance,[39] it understandably tended to look on proposals for increased benefits with a jaundiced eye.

Such proposals were, however, very numerous in 1937. One student discovered that no less than 54 bills and one proposed constitutional amendment having to do with pension liberalizations were introduced during the 1937 legislative session.[40] Under these circumstances it is not surprising that many conservatives tended to dismiss the older age groups as ungrateful complainers who were never satisfied with the state's "generosity" in providing the highest pensions in the nation but instead regarded every concession given them as a signal to demand more.

Many aged persons, however, saw the situation quite differently. To them a maximum grant of $35 a month was not altogether generous. If other states gave their old people even less, that simply revealed their niggardliness rather than California's munificence. Moreover, there were many who did not receive the maximum, because payments varied from county to county and because some pensioners had other petty sources of income.[41] Whatever allotments they did receive came only after their private affairs and those of their families had been examined in detail, a process that not only meant long delays but often strained their relationships with their families.* Equally galling was the provision allowing

* For a description of the complex administrative system for the processing of old-age pension applications, see Sam Glane, "The Administration of Public Aid to Indigent Aged in California with Special Reference to Los Angeles County" (M.S. thesis, Univ. of Southern Calif., 1937), pp. 124–28, 139–40. Early in 1937 this problem was aggravated for over 1,500 old people in Los Angeles County when the State Relief Administration, pressed for funds, dropped them

the state to take liens on pensioners' property; this aspect of the law seemed to be an attempt to force pensioners into the pauper class and to deprive them of their traditional right to transmit their property to their heirs. Finally, there were many aged persons who were ineligible to receive pensions. Some could not meet the citizenship or residence requirements; many more were over 60 but not yet 65, totally unemployed and perhaps unemployable, allegedly too old to work but legally too young to draw pensions. Thus there were many in 1937 who believed that the Old-Age Security Act needed considerable improvement.

One of these was Assemblyman John B. Pelletier from Los Angeles. An EPIC Democrat representing an area where the older age groups were dissatisfied and politically very active, Pelletier was highly sensitive to the demands of the old people and apparently genuinely interested in their welfare. On January 15, 1937, he introduced a bill to raise the maximum pension to $50 a month, lower the minimum age to 60, and eliminate both the relative-responsibility clause and the lien provision.[42] The bill produced comment throughout the state. Many feared that it would be too expensive, including the California Chamber of Commerce, which estimated that it would raise pension costs by nearly 80 per cent, and several newspapers and politicians.[43] The *EPIC News* naturally endorsed the bill strongly, and other newspapers seemed to favor it on the ground that it would at least restore California as the state with the highest pensions in the nation, a distinction that had been lost to Colorado not long before.[44] But in the end the Assembly rejected the bill, as it did a similar referendum proposal. Aside from the passage of a Welfare and Institutions Code, which merely codified existing pension and welfare statutes, and an innocuous congressional memorial calling for increased federal old-age assistance grants, there was good reason to doubt that the legislature would pass any pension legislation at all during the 1937 session.[45]

Those who doubted, however, reckoned without the skill and

---

from the relief rolls on the excuse that they had applied for old-age pensions. Their pensions were not forthcoming, however, owing to administrative delays, and they suffered acutely in the meantime. Sacramento *Union*, Mar. 6, 1937. Caught in bureaucratic tie-ups such as these, aged persons were not inclined to praise the benevolence of the Old-Age Security Act, but instead tended to react with political hostility against those who administered it.

determination of Mr. Hornblower. Pressured by the 55,000 members of the California FOE, who would soon elect him president of their organization, Hornblower apparently introduced his liberalized pension bill as much because he felt compelled to as because he wanted to.[46] Whatever his motives, he used his influence and power with such skill that he was able to steer the bill through the legislature with almost no resistance. On the first day of the session he secured 43 cosponsors for the bill in the Assembly, and with such solid initial support, all opposition crumbled. As in 1935, Hornblower finally succeeded in getting his bill passed unanimously in both houses of the legislature.[47] It was sent to Governor Merriam on the day before adjournment, and he immediately signed it even though his own citizens' conference had opposed the bill on the ground that increased pension benefits would draw hordes of aged indigents into the state.[48] The revival of this old argument seems to have served only to increase antagonisms on both sides of the pension issue.

The Hornblower Act of 1937 had considerable significance for California's aged.[49] It increased the incomes of many pensioners not by raising the amount of the grants but by curtailing deductions. Henceforth the pensioner was allowed to earn an additional income of up to $15 a month and still draw the maximum monthly pension of $35. Furthermore, the county was no longer allowed to make deductions for the rental value of property owned and occupied by the pensioner or for garden produce and other incidental commodities he might acquire. The law did establish a personal property maximum of $500 per pensioner, but so many things were excluded from this ruling, such as insurance policies and household furniture, that it was almost meaningless.

The new law, of course, was of little benefit to the really destitute pensioners, but greatly advantageous to those who were better off. Now a pensioner could own a furnished home and an insurance policy (maximum value of $1,000), raise his own vegetables, and earn $15 per month while still drawing the maximum monthly pension of $35. The penniless, propertyless, unemployed pensioner, by contrast, could draw no more than $35, and had to pay all of his expenses out of this sum. It is quite likely that after 1937 the pensioner class itself had its proletarian and aristocratic elements, so to speak, and that these divisions help to explain the mixed response of the older age groups to political movements in the state.[50]

Other provisions of the new law, however, benefited all of the aged. For example, the act allowed a pensioner to enter a hospital for temporary treatment up to 30 days without forfeiting his pension. Thus the connection between health and economic welfare among the older age groups was finally recognized by the law. More important, the legislature also eliminated a number of the features of the Old-Age Security Act that pensioners had found humiliating. The transfer provision was amended to allow a pensioner to move to any county he desired and still be certain of drawing his pension. He could move of his own volition and was no longer required to have the new county's consent to establish his residence there. This provision allowed pensioners to move to healthier locations or to be nearer friends and relatives, and many soon took advantage of it. Trivial as such a change may seem, it may have reflected at least a slight change in the public's attitude toward relief and public welfare. People seemed less bent on discouraging the aged from applying for pensions by saddling pensioners with inconveniences. Perhaps, too, they were coming to regard pensions less as a disgrace than as a way of permitting old people to live more comfortably.

The 1937 legislation also made some progress in freeing the pensioner from his supplicant status in relation to county and state welfare agencies. On the one hand, the Hornblower Act made it easier for the applicant to appeal the county's disposition of his case to the State Department of Social Welfare; on the other hand, it relieved him of excessive supervision by the latter agency by eliminating the requirement that every application approved by the county be reviewed by the state department. Furthermore, it eliminated the requirement that appeals by applicants be verified by five reputable citizens, and it forbade the counties to require paupers' oaths from the applicants. These provisions, though financially unimportant, were probably of great significance in enhancing the pensioners' self-respect.

Of even greater significance were the assaults on those twin humiliations, the relative-responsibility clause and the lien provision. Whereas previously the ability of an applicant's responsible relatives to support him, as determined by welfare officials, was enough to disqualify him from drawing a pension, now he could be disqualified only if his relatives actually supported him. In other words, the applicant now needed to show only that his relatives were not supporting him in order to make himself eligible for a pension on this count, and delinquent relatives had to be sued by the district attorney if the county wished to recover the funds paid to the pensioner. This action greatly undermined the usefulness of the relative-responsibility clause. Relatives could easily evade their responsibility in this regard, since elected district attorneys became notoriously reluctant to bring suits against local citizens who were also voters.[51]

At the same time, the new Hornblower Act deprived the counties of an even more powerful weapon against irresponsible relatives by repealing the lien provision. Heretofore, a pensioner's relatives might be motivated to support him in order to inherit his property unencumbered, but now the counties were forbidden to place liens on a pensioner's property in exchange for pensions. Thus the state simply assured delinquent relatives that they would be rewarded for their delinquency by being allowed to inherit the property of the very persons they had refused to support. This was a curious enactment. It conferred little benefit on the pensioners other than the dubious right to bequeath property, while it provided a perfect way for delinquent relatives to have their cake and eat it too.[52] The provision actually placed a premium on delinquency and for all practical purposes made the relative-responsibility clause unenforceable; it was, indeed, a legal monstrosity whereby "the liars get by and the honest get soaked," as one angry county administrator later complained.[53] Nonetheless, the new provision was popular among the aged, probably because it preserved their sense of being independent property owners.

All things considered, the relative-responsibility clause should probably have been repealed outright and the lien provision retained. The former was difficult to enforce and created severe strains in family relationships, whereas the latter was clear-cut and easily administered, and demonstrated that the state had accepted the responsibility for a pensioner's welfare. Then, too, humiliating and annoying as the lien provision was to some pensioners, it was probably emotionally satisfying to others because it gave them the feeling that they were paying their own way.[54]

Whatever the merits of the Hornblower Act of 1937, it soon proved to be both effective and expensive. Not surprisingly, then, the California public received the new law with mixed reactions. Newspaper editors and county officials praised its liberality but decried its cost. The Pasadena *Star-News*, a newspaper very sensitive to and sympathetic toward the demands of the older age groups, lauded the act as "the last word in old-age pensions," and declared that the aged were fully entitled to the increased benefits, which therefore "should not be a subject for cavil or begrudging."[55] Yet the same newspaper noted with regret that the act would probably add some 14,000 new pensioners to the rolls in Los Angeles County and increase county expenditures by some $4 million to $5 million a year.[56] "Legislators cheerfully vote more liberal allowances," the *Star-News* remarked plaintively, "and leave it to the [county] supervisors to find the money." The editor further noted with some alarm that other pension proposals were being placed on the 1938 ballot, and added, "Where the money will come from is an ever pressing query."[57]

Other counties were asking themselves the same question. Del Norte County officials expressed the fear that they would again be unable to raise the necessary pension funds by taxation, thereby jeopardizing once more the entire federal grant to the state.[58] At about the same time a Lake County grand jury advocated the elimination of many pensioners from the rolls by tightening the property requirements, and in nearby Sonoma County the supervisors petitioned the legislature to relieve the financial burden on the counties by paying a greater proportion of old-age pensions out of the general fund.[59] Soon politically powerful groups in Los Angeles and Sacramento counties also began to echo this demand for state aid to the counties, and the issue became an important one in the special session of the legislature in 1938.[60]

This session was brief, clamorous, and from the viewpoint of the older age groups, unsatisfactory. The recurrent financial crises brought on in the counties by the old-age pensions induced the spokesmen for the aged to demand that the state treasury assume more, if not all, of the pension costs being paid by the counties, and that special sources of state income be designated for this purpose. Two attempts were made to start such a system in the 1938 session, and both failed. One was a dramatic but doomed proposal by EPIC Assemblyman Ellis Patterson to put the state government in the oil business by allowing it to drill wells on its public lands and use part of the revenues to pay old-age pensions.[61] This and other colorful assaults on the oil interests, who wanted to lease these lands, were attractive to EPIC men and other liberals, but they made no headway. On the contrary, the oil bill finally passed by the 1938 legislature was precisely what Governor Merriam and the large oil companies had requested.[62]

The other attempt to secure regular state revenues for old-age pensions was a proposal to earmark a portion of the state sales tax receipts for this purpose. The Sonoma County supervisors had recommended this system, and the state senator from that county had predicted that the legislature would regard it with "considerable interest."[63] Assemblymen William Hornblower and Charles Lyon and Senator Ralph Swing were interested enough to propose investigating and studying its possibilities, but even these measures died in committee.[64]

The legislature did not adjourn, however, without giving the older age groups something. The times were too dangerous for that. The financial squeeze in the counties was so great that there were threats of tax strikes to protest the mounting cost of old-age pensions.[65] Besides exacerbating the tensions between pension groups and property owners, who after all bore the entire brunt of local taxes, these threats strengthened the hand of those demanding state aid to the counties for pension payments. Merriam, who had originally been opposed to this use of state funds, soon capitulated and agreed to request an emergency appropriation of $6 million for the counties to help defray their pension costs during the fiscal year 1938–39.[66] With the Governor's backing the deed was done; the special appropriation bill was passed by the legislature, although not without opposition.[67] Thus a more violent quarrel between the older age groups and the taxpayers' organizations was in all likelihood avoided.

Nevertheless, the older age groups were still largely dissatisfied. They felt little cause for jubilation over the emergency appropriation, which was no more than a stopgap, and whatever good will it might have won among them was more than canceled out by the grudging fashion in which it was granted. At the end of only one year the counties would probably face another financial crisis, and the old folk would once again be blamed for it. In fact, some counties continued to protest through the summer of 1938 that the large relief and pension expenditures made their budgets too high.[68] This situation gave added strength to the older age groups' demands for a pension system financed largely, if not wholly, by the state and national governments and for definite allocations of specific state revenues for this purpose.

The aged groups had other grievances. For one thing, pension allotments had decreased. The liberalizations of the Old-Age Security Act in 1937 had in effect raised the average individual monthly pension from $31.46 to $33.40 between July and September of that year, but by May 1938 the county financial crises had brought the average pension down to $32.30, where it more or less stayed for the remainder of the year.[69]

Furthermore, many aged persons were suffering from chronic deficiencies in medical care. Whether or not this situation contributed to the pension agitation of the time is difficult to determine. Certainly the general public seems to have been unaware of the problem,[70] but there is no doubt that late in 1937 it was forced on the attention of at least some citizens. Ironically, one of the most popular features of the liberalized Old-Age Security Act—the "escape hatch" from the county almshouse—was responsible for bringing the problem to light. Since 1936, it will be remembered, aged inmates of county hospitals had been allowed to apply for pensions while they were still residents there and to receive the pensions regularly as soon as they left the institution. In San Francisco nearly 300 aged inmates quickly took advantage of this provision, but soon found themselves much the worse for it. Forced to pay for food and shelter out of their miserable stipends of $35 a month or less, they found it necessary to live in slums of the worst sort. Soon the health of many who had left the San Francisco Relief Home broke down, and by December 1937 some 20 per cent had "come back to die, sick and helpless." Whereas some five out of six residents used to walk into the home, the director reported, every one of the new arrivals in the current month had been brought in on a stretcher. He also reported that one inmate had been taken out of the home by her relatives four times during the preceding year. Their custom was to wait for the home to cure her, take her out and use her pension until her health broke down again, and then commit her to the home once more. Thus a well-meaning provision in the Old-Age Security Act created a situation "entirely new . . . a public health drama without precedent" in San Francisco.[71] Just how many localities witnessed such a drama cannot be said, but it is clear that nothing whatever was done about it.

Even more distressing was a setback the older age groups received at the hands of the California Supreme Court. As we have seen, among their proudest, if also their most irrational, achievements was the repeal of the lien provision. Following through on the enactment of 1937, which prohibited the taking of liens on pensioners' property and directed the counties to release all such liens previously taken, the county of Los Angeles called upon Roger Jessup, chairman of the Board of Supervisors, to execute the necessary instruments of release. But Jessup, opposed to what he regarded as a "giveaway" program, refused to do so, and the county was forced to seek a writ of mandamus to compel him to comply. In May 1938 the California Supreme Court ruled in favor of Jessup by declaring the lien-release provision to be unconstitutional.[72] By this decision much of the work of the pension leaders was undone, and the status of pensioners as independent property owners was once again undermined.

Thus by the year 1938 the older age groups seemed to think they had grievances aplenty to publicize during the election campaign. And at this very time there was in the process of formation a new movement that was only too happy to exploit these grievances. It was called the Ham and Eggs movement.

6

Ham and Eggs

IN CALIFORNIA it was virtually raining pension plans in 1937. A number of factors probably account for this: the nationwide recession, dissatisfaction with the attitudes of the state legislature and the courts toward aged welfare proposals, newspaper opposition to old-age programs, growing public awareness of the adverse position of the older age groups, the political momentum generated by previous old-age organizations, and the promise of economic and political profits for pension promoters. Whatever the causes, there were probably at least 80 different old-age welfare schemes bidding for political support in the state during 1937 and 1938.[1] Proposals ranged all the way from large increases in old-age pension grants to free hunting and fishing licenses for those who were 65 or over. But without doubt the most sensational plan was the one hatched by a man named Robert Noble.

Noble was one of the most interesting and unprincipled men in California public life. Handsome, poised, magnetic, and highly persuasive, he made an easy living during the 1920's in Los Angeles as an inspirational radio announcer and real estate salesman.[2] His interest in swaying multitudes proved stronger than his desire to make money, however, and the 1930's found him clambering aboard the bandwagon of one mass movement after another. He enthusiastically endorsed the EPIC crusade in 1934 (a rash act that cost him his broadcasting job), but being constitutionally incapable of accepting a subordinate position in any organization, he turned against the movement, attacked its leaders, and tried to persuade its members to defect.[3] The EPIC men retaliated by publicizing some unsavory incidents in Noble's background, but by this time he was already entrenched in a California branch of the Huey Long movement.* With the collapse of this organization, he decided to give the Townsend movement a try, but was thrown out in September 1936 for using the same divisive tactics that had infuriated the EPIC leaders.[4] At this point Noble decided to found a mass movement of his own, and in these designs his unwitting ally was a respectable and rather conservative economist at Yale University named Irving Fisher.

Noble's interest in Fisher stemmed from an article Fisher had written in 1932 called "The Stamped Scrip Plan." It proposed that the United States Congress deal with the Depression by issuing an unspecified amount of a very special form of scrip money—a series of one-dollar bills with 52 spaces dated one week apart on the back.[5] Each week a two-cent postage stamp would be put in the appropriate space, and the bill would circulate at par as long as it was stamped up to date. At the end of 52 weeks all stamped bills would be redeemed at one dollar apiece, the government having by that time taken in from the sale of 52 stamps $1.04 for each bill issued. The scrip would thus be self-liquidating, and supposedly it would greatly stimulate the sale and production of goods, since people who held the money would be anxious to spend it before the next stamping date.

In this article and in a subsequent book on the subject, Fisher asserted that stamp scrip might circulate a dozen times faster than

---

* *EPIC News*, May 20, 1935. The *News* offered photographic evidence that Noble had deserted from the United States Navy and had been given a dishonorable discharge, and that he had served a prison term for robbing telephone pay stations. It also alleged that he had once been under psychiatric care; that he had been fired from a restaurant job in Pittsburgh on suspicion of robbery; that he had deserted his wife and two children, and after securing a divorce, had allowed them to become destitute while he waxed prosperous and lived with his secretary in a common-law relationship. Noble's flirtation with the Huey Long crowd ended when Long was assassinated, although Noble harvested some publicity when he attended Long's funeral and threw himself across the grave in a sensational demonstration (or impersonation) of grief. Winston and Marian Moore, *Out of the Frying Pan* (Los Angeles, 1939), p. 23; Carey McWilliams, "Ham and Eggs," *New Republic*, Oct. 25, 1939, p. 331; John H. Canterbury, " 'Ham and Eggs' in California," *The Nation*, CXLVII (1938), 408. He was also identified with William Lemke's Union Party in 1936 and in later years with a pro-Nazi organization. He was prosecuted for sedition in 1944. Los Angeles *Times*, Nov. 7, 1969; David H. Bennett, *Demagogues in the Depression* (New Brunswick, N.J., 1969), p. 247.

regular money. Thus it could serve a "pump-priming" function by "reflating" the economy and raising consumer purchasing power.[6] He also pointed out that the proposal was not a mere theorist's dream but was actually being practiced in various forms in Germany and Austria, and in dozens of communities small and large in the United States.[7] He declared that these schemes were especially useful in local welfare and make-work projects, and could become of great importance if coordinated by state governments or, better yet, completely consolidated under a national unified scrip system.[8] It should be noted, however, that Fisher was far from revolutionary in making his proposals. His article clearly pointed out that the scheme had limitations; it was not, he wrote, to be regarded as a cure-all, and would have to be supplemented by other anti-Depression policies.[9] He saw the scrip device not as a substitute for the national monetary system, but as a supplement to it, and a temporary supplement at that.[10] Furthermore, he advocated that the scrip money be issued very cautiously under controlled circumstances; the public would have to be educated to its use, and key business organizations, especially banks, would have to be persuaded to support the system.[11] The tone of these recommendations contrasts strongly with the way the scheme was promoted in California.

Whatever the plan's merits, it was bound to appeal to the imaginative Mr. Noble, who was apparently the first to tie the scrip idea to the old-age pension movement. Early in 1937 he began a series of radio broadcasts in Los Angeles extolling the merits of his New California State Pension Movement, which he later renamed the California Pension Plan.[12] This so-called movement or plan was little more than a continually repeated demand that the state issue stamp scrip in sufficient quantities to pay every unemployed person in California who was 50 or over "Twenty-Five Dollars Every Monday Morning." This slogan, without any concerted plan to carry it out, was enough to gain Noble a large following, and when he began to plead for dues-paying members to join his "organization" the response was immediate. He soon had a large following deluded into believing that they were members of an active organization with an air-tight accounting system.[13]

Then suddenly Noble found himself thrown out of his own movement by Willis and Lawrence Allen, two brothers who seem to have been louder, bolder, and even more unscrupulous than he. To recount the story of the Allen brothers' careers is a difficult task. There is a plethora of information on their activities, but most of it was written either by their violent critics or by their partisans and mouthpieces. The Allens and their associates were a controversial group, to say the least, and it is doubtful that a completely unbiased statement was ever written about any of them. According to one of the more reliable sources, Lawrence Allen, a lawyer, and Willis Allen, a former college cheerleader and hair-tonic salesman, first met Noble when they leased him office space in a building for the headquarters of his California Pension Plan.[14] They were interested in the causes of "liberal" groups like Noble's, and they conceived the idea of starting a new broadcasting station that would publicize the views of such groups in return for which the groups would place their advertising with the Cinema Advertising Agency, a corporation the Allens also controlled.[15]

At this point their actions became at least devious and possibly criminal. Having decided to open the broadcasting station in Mexico, where costs were lower, they secured the backing of George W. Berger, a California broadcasting executive. Then to gain the financial support of a Mexican businessman named M. P. Barbashano, they allegedly forged Berger's signature on a $30,000 receipt. Berger, learning of this deceit, complained to the Los Angeles police, but as luck would have it (and the Allens had a great deal), the complaint was quietly pigeonholed by a notorious police captain named Earl Kynette. Kynette, a ruthless hatchet man for the corrupt administration of the Los Angeles Mayor, Frank Shaw, had other fish to fry, and one of them was Robert Noble.[16]

Noble, in his bold, freewheeling style, had repeatedly attacked the Shaw regime over the radio, and Kynette was given the task of silencing him. Learning that Lawrence Allen was Noble's lawyer and Willis Allen his advertising manager, and that the brothers held the station contract for Noble's broadcasting time, Kynette reportedly made a deal with the Allens to eject Noble from his movement, take over the broadcasting, and divide up the profits in dues and contributions among them.[17] In September 1937 the Allens laid their plans for the putsch against Noble, and by the end of October it had been successfully carried out. In a secret meeting in Clifton's Cafeteria, a favorite rendezvous for Los Angeles "liberal" organizations, the Allens persuaded a number of

Noble's followers to defect and to reorganize the movement without him. The reconstituted board of directors consisted of the Allens, "Len" Reynolds, Fred Lenhart, William ("Pop") Burness, and a few less tractable persons who would soon be forced out and replaced by more loyal Allen men. The Allens then took over the radio broadcasts of the California Pension Plan. They opened its mail and pocketed the dues, which together with donations from Kynette enabled them to increase the activities of the movement. Noble tried to fight back, but other stations refused to sell him broadcasting time, and the public meetings he organized were broken up by Kynette's goon squads, who threw stink bombs and used other strong-arm tactics.[18] Thus the Allens gained complete control of Noble's organization and immediately began to expand its operations.

To strengthen the organization the Allens brought new henchmen to the board of directors. Some of them were relatively minor figures, such as Charles M. Hawks, a former associate of Noble's and an effective speaker, and Raymond D. Fritz, an accountant whose outspoken pro-Nazism gave the movement an anti-Semitic tinge that remained with it.[19] More important was the recruitment of Will Kindig, a one-time Los Angeles city councilman, a former EPIC functionary, and a self-styled authority on the money question.[20] Still more important was the recruitment of Sherman Bainbridge, a former EPIC official and future Townsendite who is reputed to have given the organization its nickname, Ham and Eggs, when he once shouted in a public rally, "We want our ham and eggs."[21] Bainbridge also made an important contribution to the organization when he persuaded the leaders to hire his friend, Roy G. Owens, to draw up a Ham and Eggs bill for enactment into law.[22]

The character of Roy G. Owens was a strange concoction of intelligence, mysticism, and hostility.[23] Despite his limited education (he did not finish high school), his keen intellect and varied business experience gave him a certain broad though distorted view of economic problems. He was emotionally unstable, having at one time voluntarily committed himself to a rest home, and he was attracted to weird metaphysical organizations, even to the extent of joining the Father Divine cult. When his business schemes failed and the Depression left him penniless, he responded with hostile denunciations of the economic order and with intuitive proposals to fix it. Convinced that "knowing the truth will heal any ill of the human body or the body politic," and that "economic order must be aligned with divine order for peace and security," he was impervious to any criticism of his proposals for the solution of economic ills. Owens styled himself an engineer-economist, and when the Ham and Eggs leaders gratified his ego by giving him that title, he became an undeviating spokesman for their cause.

Whatever his quirks, he served the Allens well. The first result of his labors was a complicated scrip-pension and monetary reform bill that was widely circulated and aroused much enthusiasm. At this point, however, Robert Noble staged a coup. He secured a copy of the bill and filed it with the California Secretary of State as a proposed constitutional amendment, thereby appropriating both the slogan "Twenty-Five Dollars Every Monday" and the name California Pension Plan. Owens, for his part, proved more than equal to the occasion. He drew up a new bill, the Retirement Life Payments Act, which changed the main provisions of his original bill very little but raised the proposed pension from $25 to $30 a week. Then in a master stroke he invented the slogan "Thirty Dollars Every Thursday." With that accomplished, and with the organization officially incorporated under the name Retirement Life Payments Association (RLPA), the Ham and Eggs movement was definitely launched.[24]

What was the Ham and Eggs movement? The question is hard to answer because one is never certain whether the main leaders were seriously attempting to bring about social and economic reform, whether they sought political power for its own sake, or whether they were simply engaged in a racket to make money. Whatever their motives—and probably all three were present depending on the persons involved—a few definite characteristics of the movement can be discerned: the plan on which the movement was based was an economic fantasy and could not have brought about the reforms the leaders professed it would; the organization was completely centralized and dictatorial; the methods of financial management brought considerable profit to at least some of the leaders; and the organization was amazingly adept in the arts of propaganda and in acquiring a large mass following.

The plan as Owens drew it up in 1938 had four main points. First, 30 one-dollar warrants were to be issued each week to every unemployed Californian who was 50 or over; a special two-cent state stamp would have to be placed on each warrant every Thursday. Second, a state warrant bank was to be established to sell the stamps and to facilitate the exchange of warrants; the bank would be financed by a $20 million bond issue and by the sale of $52 million worth of stock. Third, the warrants would be made legal tender for the payment of all state taxes. Fourth, a 3 per cent gross income tax would be levied on all persons and corporations in the state.[25]

The economic illiteracy of the plan was pointed out by many authorities, but probably its most effective critic was Irving Fisher himself, who resented the RLPA's travesty of his proposals.[26] Fisher pointed out that whereas his own plan called for a modest issue of scrip to supplement the existing money supply, the Ham and Eggs proposal would supplant regular money by making scrip far more plentiful than federal currency. As a result most banks and businesses would refuse to accept the scrip, and it would circulate only at a heavy discount.[27] Others pointed out that in these circumstances the state, having promised to accept the depreciated scrip in taxes, would be in danger of bankruptcy.[28]

Whatever the movement lacked in academic sophistication it made up for in organization. By the end of 1938 it had local representatives in 33 counties, including all of the most populous ones; by March 1939 it had representatives in every county except sparsely populated Mono County.[29] Even these representatives, however, to say nothing of the rank and file, had no voice in the organization's affairs. Local meetings and rallies were not held under the auspices of local clubs, as in the Townsend movement, but were called by speakers sent out from the Ham and Eggs headquarters in Los Angeles. The speakers, moreover, were closely controlled by the board of directors, which in the final analysis seems to have been controlled by Willis and Lawrence Allen.[30] The Ham and Eggs movement, then, presents a classic case of deviant leadership. Deprived of responsible roles within the organization, its masses of aged members were unable to develop their own leaders and instead found themselves utterly dependent on the Allens and their associates, who were willing to endure the social stigma of advocating an unpopular and disreputable cause supposedly on the members' behalf.

As usual, the leaders were able to extract rather high prices for these services. One of the most noticeable aspects of the entire movement was the leaders' unceasing appeal for funds. Besides the dues of a penny a day, members were urged to buy Ham and Eggs booklets, copies of the Ham and Eggs proposal, lapel buttons, and the like, and to patronize many promotional road shows and other vote-getting entertainments that were always calculated to at least pay their own costs.[31] By such means an admitted $332,000 was brought into the RLPA treasury in 1938 and more than $590,000 in 1939.[32] Although the Allens claimed that all of these receipts were paid out again in promotion costs and that no one in the organization received a salary of more than $30 a week,[33] their own accounting shows clearly that these promotion expenditures were paid mainly into corporations the Allens owned, such as their Cinema Advertising Agency.* Under this type of *crédit mobilier* arrangement, the profits derived from handling Ham and Eggs promotional ventures were no doubt substantial.

However blatantly the Ham and Eggs leaders exploited the movement, they seemed to have no trouble attracting followers. Totally uninhibited in promoting their plan in the press and over the radio, and highly skillful in playing on the economic and social frustrations of the aged and down-and-out, Ham and Eggs leaders acquired a formidable mass following in a relatively short time. By the end of 1938 they claimed some 270,000 members and over a million supporters, and by October 1939 their membership had allegedly grown to some 362,000.[34] With so many followers, they were in a strong position to exert considerable sway in the California political arena.

The leaders were not reluctant to use this strength. Throughout the summer of 1938 California was the scene of innumerable Ham and Eggs rallies, the attendance at which, especially in southern California, often ran into the thousands.[35] A mixture of Midwestern folksiness, revivalistic enthusiasm, hostility toward the existing

---

* *National Ham and Eggs*, Oct. 14, 1939. According to the Moores it was the former shellac merchant Raymond Fritz who masterminded these bookkeeping procedures. They also claimed that when money began to pour into Ham and Eggs headquarters Willis Allen paced up and down the office chuckling "Is she sweet or is she sweet? Wowie!" Winston and Marian Moore, *Out of the Frying Pan* (Los Angeles, 1939), pp. 67, 69–70, 98–99.

order, and general bewilderment seemed to dominate these affairs. According to one newspaper article: "They open each meeting with a choir-like verse of Halleluiah. En masse they stand with outstretched arms and pledge allegiance to the giant American flag on the platform, and business is never taken up before the party cheer—'5-10-15-20-25-30-Thursday'—is yelled fervently by 2,500 or more voices." Although "an atmosphere of homeyness" and "a feeling of good fellowship" were noticeable traits at these meetings, the article continued, the members were quick to brand opponents of the Ham and Eggs plan as tools of "vested interests" and "greed mongers." And the speakers were able to instill in the followers a blind faith in the efficacy of the plan, even when they admitted that they could not answer some embarrassing questions raised about it. "The answer to that will be worked out later," was the reply given to many such questions, and the audience seemed to find this response perfectly acceptable.[36]

Typical of the Ham and Eggs style of campaigning was the Archie Price incident. Price was a 62-year-old pauper who had committed suicide in a San Diego public park and had left behind a note reading "Too young to receive an old-age pension and too old to find work." Seizing on Price's death as a dramatic demonstration that their cause was just, the Ham and Eggs leaders led a gigantic procession to San Diego. They had Price's corpse exhumed from the potter's field and reinterred in an upper-class cemetery, while emotional funeral orations were preached over loudspeakers to an estimated 7,000 overwrought Ham and Eggers. The star of this ghoulish show was none other than Sheridan Downey, candidate for United States Senator and in the process of becoming closely associated with the Ham and Eggs cause. At his eloquent best Downey admonished his listeners to think of Price as a martyr who had died for a sacred cause, "the right of senior citizens to dignity, to security, to life."[37]

With such catchy promotional schemes as these, the leaders sought to generate enthusiasm for their Ham and Eggs amendment. At the same time an army of RLPA workers was quietly soliciting petition signatures to qualify the proposed amendment on the November ballot. In midsummer the general public, and especially the business community, was astounded to learn that the measure had qualified with an unheard-of 789,000 signatures.[38]

This demonstration of power gave the Ham and Eggers some leverage with candidates for public office, especially with Democrats, who being perennially out of power could not afford to reject any offers of political support.[39]

Not surprisingly, then, the Ham and Eggs issue figured prominently in the Democratic gubernatorial race. Two of the five main contenders in the primary, Herbert C. Legg and William H. Neblett, were dark horses and did not commit themselves on the Ham and Eggs issue. However, Daniel C. Murphy, whose old-age pension record was excellent, took a courageous stand against Ham and Eggs, a stand that was probably responsible for his losing the race.[40] The conservative John F. Dockweiler and the liberal Culbert L. Olson remained as the chief contenders. Dockweiler quickly endorsed the Ham and Eggs initiative and almost received the Allen brothers' endorsement as a result.[41] Olson at first tried to campaign on his well-established pro-pension record and on his efforts to keep the Ham and Eggs proposal on the ballot (there was talk of disqualifying it on technicalities) in order to give it a fair trial before the voters. In the middle of August, however, he succumbed and sent two telegrams to RLPA headquarters strongly endorsing the initiative.[42] Although he was later to regret this decision, it was probably instrumental in winning him the election.

The Ham and Eggs issue was probably also decisive in the Democratic primaries for United States senator and lieutenant governor.* In the former race Sheridan Downey, who had the fervent though unofficial backing of Ham and Eggs plus the support of the Townsendites, of the remnants of EPIC, and of a militant minority of the regular Democratic Party, decisively defeated the incumbent, William Gibbs McAdoo, even though McAdoo had the open support of President Roosevelt. The President, furthermore, had attacked "those who advocate shortcuts to utopia or fantastic financial schemes."[43] In the canvass for the nomination for lieutenant governor, the outspoken EPIC Assemblyman Ellis Patterson defeated a field of opponents after having endorsed the

---

* Interestingly enough, however, the Ham and Eggs organization did not officially endorse any of the winning candidates. In fact, the only candidate it endorsed, Earl S. Kegley for attorney general, lost heavily to Earl Warren. Los Angeles County Democratic Slate, in Bancroft Library Collection of Campaign Literature from the California Election of 1938, University of California, Berkeley; State of California, Secretary of State, *Statement of Vote*, Primary Election, Aug. 30, 1938, pp. 18–19.

Ham and Eggs program.[44] All things considered, the results of the primary seemed to indicate that the Ham and Eggs movement was a force to be reckoned with in the general election.

After the primary, the Ham and Eggs organization continued to make its sensational appeals and promises to the voters,[45] but now a formidable, if belated, opposition began to develop. Not only did the state Chamber of Commerce raise a campaign fund to oppose Ham and Eggs,[46] but a number of banks and insurance companies declared that they could not legally handle Ham and Eggs warrants, and they were at least partly upheld in this opinion by the state Attorney General.[47] Many state employees and public school teachers launched a massive assault against the proposal because they feared that they would be forced to accept their salaries in depreciated scrip.[48] Eight Stanford University economists and sociologists published a statement attacking the plan.[49] The Townsendites, apparently resentful of Ham and Eggs competition for pension support, criticized the plan in a fashion that was surprisingly sophisticated in view of the economic naïveté of their own scheme.[50] Finally, the newspapers of the state were almost unanimously opposed to the plan, despite the fact that many of their readers strongly supported it. Such a battery of opposition began to make the adoption of the Ham and Eggs amendment seem less certain as the election drew near.

It was one thing for certain groups to oppose the initiative, but it was quite another thing for the candidates to do so. Sheridan Downey continued to woo the support of the Ham and Eggers not only by endorsing their program but by joining them in opposing a conservative anti-picketing measure that was also on the ballot.[51] This stand brought him additional support from organized labor that, combined with an explicit endorsement from President Roosevelt, made his victory over the stodgy Republican candidate, Philip Bancroft, seem certain.[52]

In the race for governor a curious situation developed. The Democrats feared that Olson's endorsement of the Ham and Eggs program would split the party, since many northern Californians were violently opposed to it. Surprisingly, however, Willis Allen rescued them from the dilemma at the party convention by asking them to avoid discussing the issue, which he said transcended party lines.[53] The Democrats were only too delighted to comply with this request, and as a result the Ham and Eggs issue was played down somewhat throughout the rest of the gubernatorial campaign. Surprisingly, too, when Olson wavered on the issue,[54] the Allens toyed with the idea of endorsing the Republican candidate, incumbent Frank Merriam, even though he had taken a strong stand against the Ham and Eggs scheme.[55] It is difficult to understand why the Allens would deliberately dissipate their political support in this manner unless they were trying to lose the election. After all, the "golden stream" of contributions would dry up if the Ham and Eggs measure was enacted, and the Ham and Eggs leaders would be left with the task of trying to make their monstrosity work.

The Allens faced an even greater embarrassment at this time from their former colleague, the irrepressible Robert Noble. He had cleverly filed for governor on the Commonwealth Party ticket, and having no opposition, had become a bona fide contender by securing a mere 274 votes.[56] At first he offered to help the Allens secure the passage of the Ham and Eggs amendment, provided they would support his candidacy and acknowledge him as the founder of the movement.[57] The Allens turned a deaf ear to his overtures, however, and when Len Reynolds of the Ham and Eggs board of directors bloodied Noble's nose as he tried to enter a public Ham and Eggs meeting, he decided to expose the organization.[58] He began to make radio broadcasts telling of the Allens' collusion with the corrupt Mayor Shaw, who had since been recalled, and of their dealings with Earl Kynette, who had since been sent to prison for attempted murder.[59] Apparently Kynette then decided to use the occasion to take his own revenge. He brought suit against the Allens for failing to give him his third of the Ham and Eggs profits, and he also revealed the whereabouts of the document forged by the Allens to George Berger, who accordingly charged the Allens with forgery. Although both charges were eventually dismissed, they must have sounded incriminating enough at the time.[60]

These developments, however, hardly seemed to bother the Allens at all. When one of the officials of the Ham and Eggs movement asked the Allens to resign because they might hurt the movement's chances in the election, they not only refused but seemed to shrug off the importance of winning. Indeed, during the last week of the campaign when Noble's sensational disclosures were being made and Kynette's law suit was being filed, the Allens al-

legedly spent less money in campaigning than before, even though
Sherman Bainbridge urged them to "shoot the works." Again it
seems plausible that the Allens were trying to lose the election in
order to keep contributions flowing in. They reportedly told Bainbridge, in fact, that they were saving money to finance their activities *after* the election.[61]

The outcome of the election was victory for the Ham and Eggs
candidates (Downey, Olson, and Patterson) and a fairly narrow
defeat for the Ham and Eggs initiative by a vote of 1,143,670 to
1,398,999.[62] With a vote this close it was easy for the Ham and Eggs
leaders to sustain the enthusiasm of the rank and file and to continue gathering support for their "reforms." Indeed, after their
election defeat the Ham and Eggers seemed stronger than ever. On
November 13, 1938, the first Sunday after the election, they held
a rally in the Shrine Auditorium in Los Angeles. The meeting was
attended by some 8,000 people who responded deafeningly when
asked if they wanted to try again, and who reportedly contributed
$1,700 to get the new campaign started.[63]

Shortly afterward, in the first issue of the movement's new newspaper, *National Ham and Eggs*, the board of directors affirmed in
ringing tones its "unswerving determination to stand firm" despite
the bankers who, they charged, were "trying to destroy the power
of this organization."[64] This statement set the tone for all subsequent Ham and Eggs propaganda—barrages of populistic denunciations of bankers and so-called monopolies combined with an
unrestrained use of superlatives in promoting Ham and Eggs proposals. In the same issue the editors called the recent election only
the first battle against "our iniquitous money system and the legal-
ized racketeers who operate it," and declared that they would
"never be able to dethrone the dollar dynasty" until they could
"make all the people understand its hellish character." To perform this task, the leaders announced that they would circulate
a gigantic new petition requesting the governor to call a new election in 1939 so that the people could vote once more on a Ham
and Eggs amendment.

In the process of launching this new (and profitable) campaign,
the Allens found it necessary to do a certain amount of rebuilding
in the movement. First they had to eliminate internal opposition,
and this they did in a smooth and ruthless fashion. A number of
the Ham and Eggs officials, led by Sherman Bainbridge, continued

to oppose the Allens because of their unsavory past and their refusal to stop taking profits from the organization through the Cinema Advertising Agency. With their firm control over the organization and its propaganda outlets, the Allens forced Bainbridge and his followers out of the organization and then attacked them for having "sold out" to the "interests."[65]

Another task before the Allens was to tighten and streamline the state organization. The movement had grown so fast and the California population was always in such a state of flux that to perfect an efficient statewide political apparatus would seem to have been almost impossible. Luckily, however, the Allens found in George McLain the right man for the job. McLain, who later became the dominant pension leader in the state, had participated unsuccessfully in various political reform movements in Los Angeles since the start of the Depression; he had become especially hostile toward the state old-age pension system because of indignities he felt had been inflicted on his father by pension administrators.[66] Hired by the Ham and Eggs board as a district manager in December 1938, McLain proved himself not only "a hell of a hard worker," as one RLPA official observed, but also a genius at organization.[67]

McLain divided the state into congressional districts headed by district coordinators; these were in turn divided into assembly districts headed by district managers; assembly districts were each divided into ten sections headed by section supervisors; and each section was divided into ten precincts headed by a precinct captain and four assistants. Once this network was set up, the orders of the board of directors could be sent out by bulletin or telephone with the assurance that they would be relayed down to the grassroots level very quickly.[68] These techniques and the unrestrained use of propaganda were a resounding success in increasing the organization's membership. By midsummer there were apparently well over 300,000 members, with new members joining at the rate of 600 a day; the circulation of *National Ham and Eggs,* by now a 28-page publication with more than seven pages of advertising, was between 60,000 and 100,000; and the income of the organization was said to average some $55,000 a month.[69] Thus the Ham and Eggs leaders were in a strong position to create a stir on the California political scene in 1939.

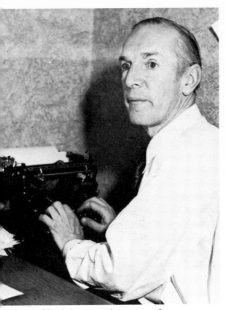

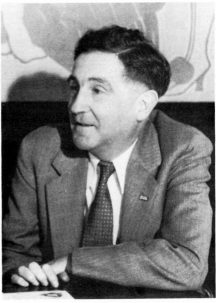

1. Upton Sinclair at work on copy for
EPIC News, September 1934

2. Sheridan Downey, Sinclair's running mate

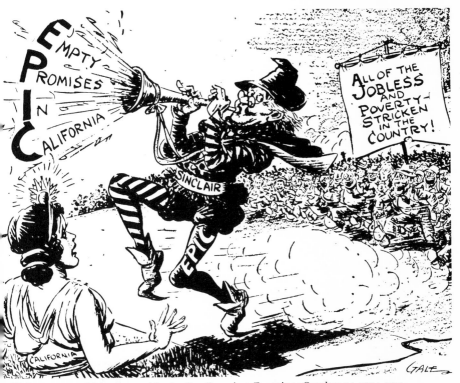

3. This cartoon, which appeared in the *San Francisco Examiner* October 24, 1934, was
one of a series that began in the newspaper on October 23 and continued
daily through the eve of the election, November 4.

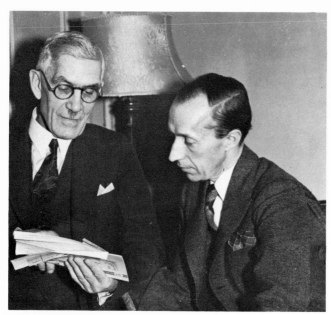

4. Dr. Francis E. Townsend (left) with Robert E. Clements, national secretary of the Townsend movement, at a meeting in New York, February 5, 1935

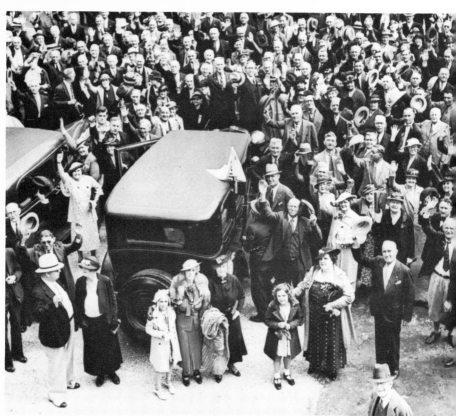

5. Washington-bound caravan leaving Los Angeles on May 6, 1936, with petitions demanding that Congress enact the major points of the Townsend Plan

One of the many well-attended Townsend rallies. This one, staged at Pasadena's Rose Bowl in 1936, drew some 15,000 persons.

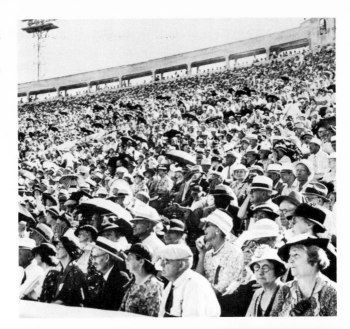

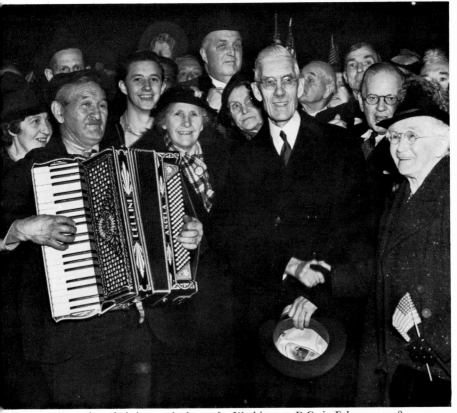

7. Townsendites salute their hero as he leaves for Washington, D.C., in February 1938 to serve a 30-day jail sentence for refusing to testify before a House committee.

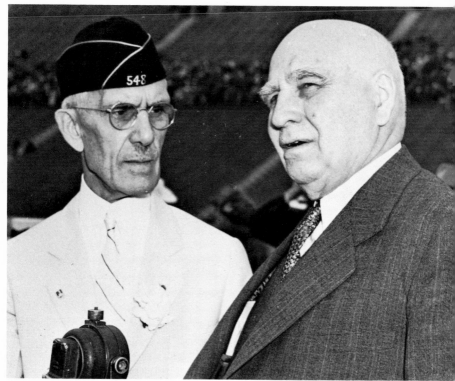

8. Gov. Frank E. Merriam (right) joining Townsend to help open the Townsend Plan's third annual convention. Held in the Los Angeles Coliseum June 20–23, 1938, the convention was attended by some 20,000 persons from all over the country.

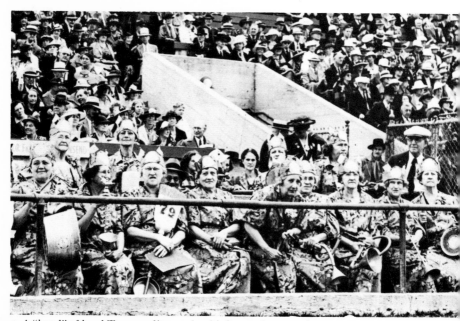

9. A "band" of loyal Townsendites at the third annual convention

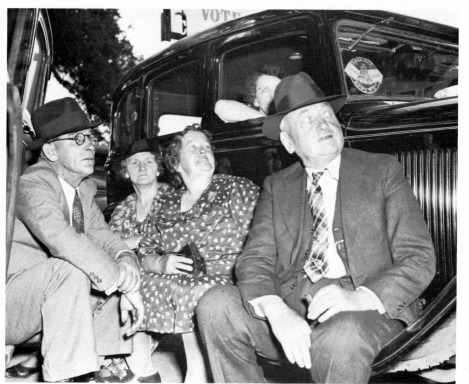

10. Ham and Egg boosters at rally in Sunland, Calif., October 9, 1938. Speaker was Sherman Bainbridge, former member of the EPIC Board of Directors who became active in the Ham and Eggs movement.

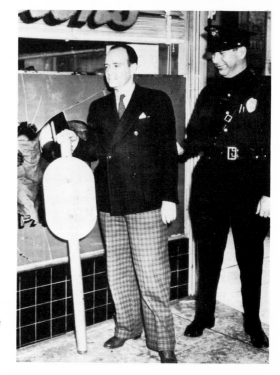

11. Robert Noble, still holding the "No Left Turn" sign he used to smash the window of an auto loan company, is taken into custody. The incident took place on December 7, 1938. Noble charged that the company, which had sponsored his radio broadcasts, had cut him off the air without notice.

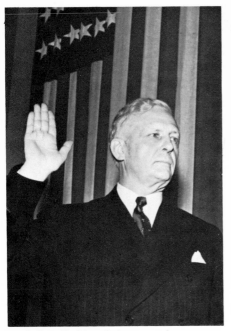

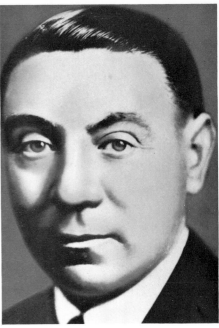

12. Culbert L. Olson being sworn in as Governor, January 2, 1939

13. California Assemblyman William B. Hornblower

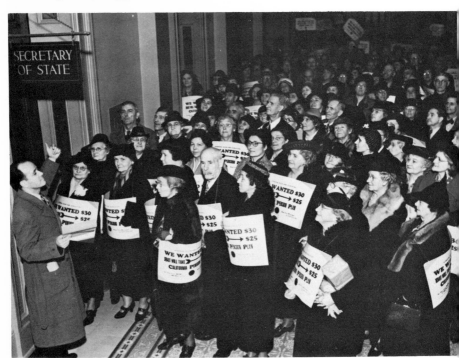

14. Led by Robert Noble, picketers descend on State Capitol in Sacramento to threaten Governor Olson with a recall movement if he does not have pension laws enacted. Olson was making his inaugural address at the time.

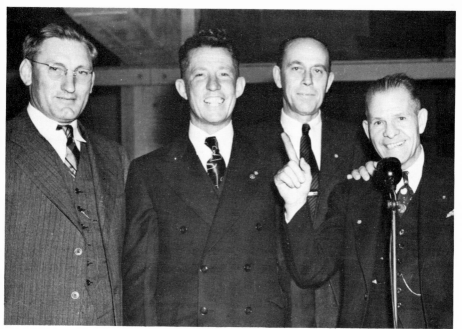

15. At Los Angeles Shrine Auditorium, November 5, 1939: (left to right) Lt. Gov. Ellis Patterson, with Lawrence W. Allen, Roy G. Owens, and William R. Peeler of the Ham and Eggs movement

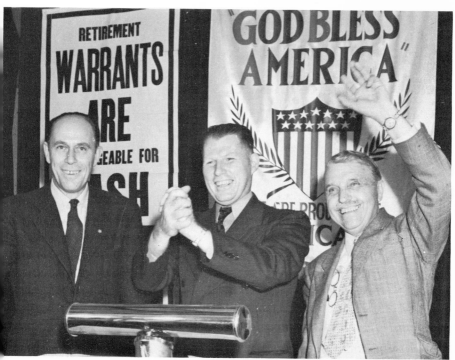

6. (Left to right) Roy G. Owens, Willis Allen, and Will H. Kindig in their main Los Angeles campaign headquarters on the night of November 6, 1939, the eve of the election in which their "$30-Every-Thursday" plan was rejected by California voters

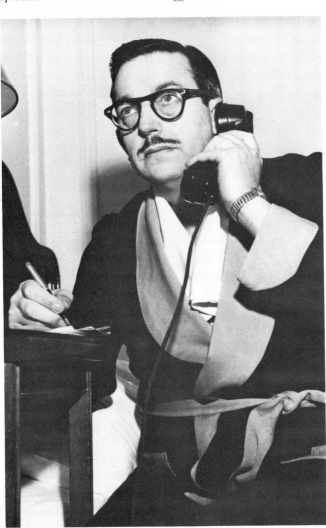

NATIONAL

Ham and Eggs

5¢   5¢

Life Begins at 50

RETIREMENT   **LIFE PAYMENTS**   ASSOCIATION

$30 A WEEK for life

☆   ☆

National Campaign Committee

6TH N. HIGHLAND AVE.· HOLLYWOOD, CAL.

$30 EVERY Thursday

VOLUME 1   —6   LOS ANGELES   SATURDAY, OCTOBER 21, 1939   SAN FRANCISCO   NUMBER 47

17. Masthead of *National Ham and Eggs*

18. George McLain, founder of the California
League of Senior Citizens

In late December the leaders unveiled the new Ham and Eggs initiative amendment. It was a complicated Rube Goldberg contraption, open to what were by now the standard objections that it would be unworkable and could lead to state bankruptcy, as well as to charges that it amounted to regressive taxation and financial and political dictatorship.[70] The proposal included the familiar "Thirty Thursday" stamp scrip scheme; a so-called credit clearings bank, which was to be a state monopoly doing business in both scrip and money; a 3 percent "gross receipts tax" on all transactions made in money but not in scrip; and the appointment of either Roy Owens or Will Kindig to be a state "administrator," with absolute control over the new monetary system, unfettered by either state officials or the courts. The initiative was the brainchild of Roy Owens, who quite obviously dreamed of enacting the measure into law and ruling benevolently over the new financial order it would create.

More striking than the initiative itself was the unbridled ballyhoo that accompanied it. "We have really dated a miracle this time," Owens modestly remarked as he finished drafting the measure, which *National Ham and Eggs* billed in its December 24 issue as a "surprise Christmas package . . . offering the greatest challenge ever faced by the present financial dynasty." Later the paper described the program as "unprecedented in the annals of American economic life," and as "the Nation's No. 1 economic campaign— the trail blazing precedent smashing Retirement Life Payments Act to bring $30 a Week For Life to California Senior Citizens."[71] Perhaps the best sample of the Ham and Eggs rhetoric, however, is the editorial from the December 24 issue, entitled "Christmas Beacon of 1938":

This day, 1938 years ago, there appeared a star, the light of which predicted that the brotherhood of men is the only doctrine that can bring welfare, happiness and tranquillity to humanity.

It took 1938 years before the rays from that star succeeded in igniting a beacon on this earth, from which radiates the right understanding of how to give that doctrine a practical working form.

That beacon is now blazing in California and is known to the world as "Ham and Eggs." . . .

The beacon named itself with no high flown words, or fancy phrases, but chose the three simple words "Ham and Eggs" because every individual, humble or otherwise, will instantly grasp the significance thereof.

Every man knows that a daily breakfast similar to that described by those three words will give him the strength, health and vigor to begin his everyday pursuit of bringing about welfare, tranquillity and happiness into the homes of those he loves.

The rays of that star of 1938 years ago also announced the coming of the Christ-man of that time, whose only exhibit of wrath, while on earth, expressed itself by whipping the money demagogues from the steps leading up to that temple which enshrines the welfare, happiness and tranquillity, which God ordained for humanity at large.

True to the methods practiced by the money demagogues of ancient times, who that time crucified the Redeemer, the money demagogues of today, led by the international bankers, ruthlessly endeavor to crucify every people's movement, which can bring peace and contentment to humanity, and the viciousness with which they have fought against "Ham and Eggs" becoming enacted into law shows clearly their understanding that the principles involved in "Ham and Eggs" will eradicate their practices and bring peace and tranquillity to humanity, besides shearing the international bankers of their God-forsaken methods to hold humanity in methodical economic slavery.[72]

If such methods were tasteless and vaguely anti-Semitic, they were also extremely effective. With their organization functioning smoothly and with mass enthusiasm running high, the Ham and Eggs leaders inaugurated a massive petition-circulating campaign, complete with constant appeals for contributions in labor and money to sustain it.* Soon mass meetings were being held all over the state, and the Ham and Eggers made concerted and often successful appeals to gain the support of labor unions and small businessmen in their petition drives.[73] It was evident that Ham and Eggs was gaining adherents not only among the aged and the lower classes, but among many sectors of the middle class as well.[74]

The success of this new drive was soon apparent. With their petition-circulating techniques refined to a science by McLain, the Ham and Eggs leaders were able to present the Secretary of State

* *National Ham and Eggs*, Jan. 21, 1939. A typical appeal for funds was made in the same issue: "What we must have is money to get these petitions printed. ...All that remains is for you to stop for a minute and think about what thirty dollars a week for life means to you. Then get in and do your part." This materialistic theme was repeated in an anonymous poem in the February 18 issue, the last stanza of which read:

> Let's stay away from politics
> Regardless of who hollers
> Let's not be fooled by childish tricks
> LET'S GET OUR THIRTY DOLLARS

with nearly 400,000 signed petitions in almost no time; further-more, they promised the Governor a million signatures before their drive was ended.[75] Clearly the next move was up to Governor Olson, and just as clearly the Governor would face a storm of re-sentment from one side or the other whether he granted or refused the Allens' demand for a special election. In the end Olson proved more than equal to the occasion. He found a way to grant the Ham and Eggers' request, and at the same time to ensure their defeat.

At first it seemed as though Governor Olson and the RLPA were on a honeymoon. In an official editorial two weeks before Olson's inauguration the Ham and Eggs leaders declared, "We are in fullest sympathy with Governor Olson."[76] The Governor want-ed pension increases, they explained, but with the already high budget deficit any attempt to finance increases "under the taxation system" would "bring ruin to the home owner and the business man." In this and subsequent editorials, to be sure, the Ham and Eggs leaders supported Olson's tax and reform policies; but they also cleverly implied that their plan would achieve such reforms and solve all fiscal problems without increasing taxes on the middle and upper classes and without disturbing the status quo.[77] The Ham and Eggs strategy in the early months of 1939 was to woo Olson and induce him to call a special election for the Ham and Eggs amendment, and at the same time to generate mass public support for the amendment as a great social cure-all.

In line with this strategy, and for other reasons, *National Ham and Eggs* looked with austere disdain on Robert Noble's next caper. That ubiquitous rabble-rouser organized a spectacular march to Sacramento on inauguration day to demand that Olson "keep his promises" regarding old-age pensions. The marchers carried placards reading "$25 Every Monday Morning," "Pensions, Governor! Not Phony Promises!" "We Wanted $30 But Will Take $25," "We Want Action Now, or Recall For You," "Keep Your Promises or Out You Go," and "If We're Heading For Utopia, Why Not Short Cuts?"[78] At the inauguration ceremony Noble brashly attempted to disrupt the proceedings and was ejected by the police.[79] *National Ham and Eggs* naturally condemned the whole affair, no doubt with great glee: "Such childish methods will never win thinking people to our cause, so our job is to con-tinue to conduct a clean, orderly campaign and refrain from per-mitting ourselves to be linked to these silly excursions."[80] Perhaps the most remarkable of Noble's achievements was to make Ham and Eggs appear respectable by comparison.

The Ham and Eggers did not confine themselves, however, to toasting the Governor's health. They subjected him to unremitting pressure to call a special election. They proceeded at full speed with their petition drive and staged innumerable mass rallies that invariably ended in direct appeals to the Governor to grant their wish. The pressure became intense when public officials like Lieutenant Governor Patterson and Nathan T. Porter, one of Olson's administrative aides, appeared at Ham and Eggs rallies and fervently endorsed the proposed initiative, assuring the audiences that Olson would accede to their request.[81] At first Olson withstood the pressure, concentrating his efforts instead on his legislative program of reform, which was already in deep trouble. But when the Allens announced that they had filed more than a half-million petition signatures and planned to present the Governor with another 600,000 at a mass rally in Sacramento, he apparently made up his mind to capitulate.[82]

On May 18 thousands of Ham and Eggers descended on the capitol bearing bundles of petitions like trophies of war.[83] Receiving a delegation led by Willis Allen, Olson stated that he was "inclined to respond to these petitions and call a special election," and then, succumbing to further pressure, he attended the Ham and Eggs rally at the fair grounds that evening and formally announced that he would call for the election.[84] Although his announcement was received with wild enthusiasm, there was less jubilation over his closing remark: "I am in sympathy with the objectives of your plan, but I not do want you to infer that I believe in the feasibility of the plan or that it would accomplish these objectives if adopted."[85] It may also have been disturbing to some that Olson did not set a date for the election. Instead he said the election would be "at the earliest possible moment" and assured the Ham and Eggers that they would be "entirely satisfied" with his decision.[86] Since the Allens had already made known their desire that the election be held by August 15, 1939,[87] when Ham and Eggs enthusiasm would supposedly be at its crest, both friends and foes began to prepare themselves for a midsummer election.

As a result of Olson's capitulation, California became in 1939 the scene of an election campaign rivaling in bitterness the Sinclair campaign of five years before. Unlike the 1934 election, however, this was no contest between liberals and conservatives or revolutionaries and reactionaries, for many of the liberal-labor-intellectual groups that had supported Sinclair in 1934 now cooperated closely with moderate and conservative groups to defeat Ham and Eggs. Among the amendment's more moderate opponents there were probably many who were less repelled by its contents than by the patent insincerity, the strident hucksterism, and the hardbreathing press agentry with which it was forced on them. Matters of taste, as we have seen, were no consideration to the Ham and Eggs leaders. And if many of them, unlike Owens, seemed flagrantly insincere in professing to believe in their program, they seemed this time in dead earnest about using the program to gain political power for sinister ends. "Never has more drooling drivel poured forth from the mouths of campaign leaders than that coming from these self-appointed saviors—Owens, Kindig, Allen, etc.," snarled one infuriated newspaper editor; "democratic government itself is threatened by a frank attempt to establish dictatorship in the guise of a pension plan."[88]

The California press, a press that was "kept" by bankers and businessmen, according to *National Ham and Eggs*, spearheaded the opposition.[89] It continually hammered away at the unsoundness of the warrant system and the dictatorial aspect of the provision whereby Roy Owens was to become the unchallenged fiscal arbiter of the state.[90] The California Bankers' Association also specifically opposed the measure, declaring that it would impair the state's financial soundness. This opposition, however, was welcomed by the Ham and Eggs leaders, who had long since been calling bankers "public enemy number one," "loan rangers," and the like.* An example of their intense anti-banker rhetoric is afforded by the following excerpt from a speech by Roy Owens:

* *National Ham and Eggs*, June 3, 1939, Dec. 3, 1938. An interesting sidelight of this feud was the warrant crisis of 1939, in which the state government was unable for a time to market its tax anticipation warrants and was threatened with insolvency. The bankers declared that the state's plight had been caused by uncertainty about the state's fiscal soundness, caused in turn by the threat that the Ham and Eggs amendment might pass. The Ham and Eggs leaders charged, for their part, that the crisis was deliberately fomented by the bankers to make money and to undermine confidence in Ham and Eggs. *Ibid.*, Aug. 5, Sept. 16, Sept. 23, 1939; Bakersfield *Californian*, Sept. 19, 1939; Pasadena *Star-News*, Sept. 20, 1939.

They say that we've never been the head of a bank. . . . And we haven't!
They say we've never been the head of any big corporation. . . . And we
haven't!
They say we were on WPA. . . . And we were!
They say we've never handled large sums of money. . . . And we haven't!
But we're going to handle them and you can tell that to your bankers!
They say this tax is only a subterfuge to drive bankers' money out of
the market. . . . And it is!
They say that it will shake the financial structure of the world. . . . And
it will!
They call us crackpots. . . . And we are! We're going to crack their pots
wide open![91]

More formidable opposition to Ham and Eggs came from citizens' committees led by such prominent personages as James K. Lytle, President of the California Congress of Parents and Teachers; former Governor George C. Pardee; former Attorney General U. S. Webb; and 138 economists from leading California colleges and universities.[92] Other opposition came from certain sectors of organized labor, which feared the measure would jeopardize their right to picket; from state employees and schoolteachers, who again feared for their salaries; from other pension leaders, like Sinclair, Townsend, and Noble; and from various individuals who brought lawsuits against the Allens and other Ham and Eggs leaders.[93]

But in the last analysis the RLPA's greatest foe turned out to be Governor Olson. The Governor had been exhibiting a growing coolness toward Ham and Eggs since his announcement of the special election, and when he began to say that his only reason for calling it was to dispose of the issue before the election of 1940, the Ham and Eggers began to show considerable concern.[94] Declaring that the legislature was wrecking Olson's version of the New Deal, which was true enough, and that Olson's only chance to obtain real reform in California was to stick with his "friends" in the Ham and Eggs movement, they demanded that he quickly proclaim August 15 the election date.[95] On July 1, however, to the utter chagrin of the Ham and Eggers, Olson announced that the election would take place on November 7, a date that would come long after the Ham and Eggs popularity had reached its peak, and one that provided plenty of time for the opposition to gather its strength.[96]

The Ham and Eggs leadership was furious at what they saw as Olson's betrayal. In the first issue of the party newspaper after the Governor's announcement the editors printed the two telegrams in which Olson had endorsed Ham and Eggs in the primary election of 1938. Then they declared that he had "turned his back on the only friends he ever had," in choosing to "listen and be guided by the reactionary element."[97] But the leaders stoutly resisted all proposals to institute a recall campaign against Olson, saying that such a move would dissipate their energies at a time when they needed greater concentration of effort to secure the passage of their amendment.[98] They did, however, succeed in persuading Lieutenant Governor Patterson and the Governor's administrative aide, Nathan T. Porter to defect completely from Olson's side to theirs.* The vociferous support these former associates gave to the movement doubtless caused Olson considerable embarrassment.

Olson fought back with weapons of his own. In announcing the special election he questioned the constitutionality of the Ham and Eggs proposal and stated: "I would be false to my own conscience and sense of duty if I failed to here express my belief that if adopted, this measure would fail to achieve its objectives, would disappoint the hopes of its supporters, and would retard instead of aid our progress to a better economic order."[99] When the San Francisco *News* published this statement in an anti–Ham and Eggs advertisement, Olson at first protested the "unauthorized" use of his name and photograph in a highly conservative newspaper; later, however, he promoted George Killion, the member of his staff responsible for the advertisement, to a higher position.[100]

Under Olson's leadership, or at least with his knowledge and tacit assent, officials of a number of state executive agencies became active opponents of Ham and Eggs. The State Director of Finance, John R. Richards, and the State Superintendent of Banks, E. W. Wilson, predicted economic ruin if the measure passed, while Willis Allen complained that employees in the State Relief Admin-

---

* *National Ham and Eggs,* July 22, Aug. 26, Sept. 30, 1939; San Francisco *Chronicle,* July 3, July 15, 1939. At first Patterson tried to hold the Ham and Eggers' loyalty to Olson, advising them to "stay with your Governor" at a Fourth of July Ham and Eggs rally in Los Angeles. But when they responded by singing "Goodby, Olson, we're going to leave you now," Patterson went along with them and became thereafter an outspoken advocate of the Ham and Eggs plan. Pasadena *Star-News,* July 7, 1939.

istration and in the Department of Public Works were openly engaged in anti–Ham and Eggs political activity.[101] The Secretary of State demanded a more rigid accounting of political campaign funds spent by the Ham and Eggs organization, and the Social Welfare Board declared that the passage of the scrip scheme would make the state ineligible to receive any more federal funds from the Social Security Administration—a telling blow to the Ham and Eggers, even if the board's interpretation of the Social Security Act was doubtful.[102] Olson's floor leader in the state Senate, Robert W. Kenny, was an outspoken opponent of the measure, as were, of course, many legislators who were enemies of the Governor.[103] Finally, Olson himself came out strongly against the amendment, particularly in an effective speech on November 5.[104]

The Ham and Eggers, meanwhile, were undertaking vigorous measures of their own. They sought very strenuously to gain the support of such groups as laborers, Negroes, and liberal elements in the Democratic Party, and they stepped up the number and intensity of their mass meetings and other entertainments.[105] They also perfected their organized campaign to get out the vote, and in a flagrantly dishonest attempt to make the proposal more attractive, they suddenly announced that Ham and Eggs warrants would be redeemable at face value in United States currency after being in circulation not for 52 weeks but for only 30 days![106] It is easy to agree with a newspaper editor who described this move as

proof of deliberate deception on the part of Ham and Eggs propagandists. To pay $1 cash for a warrant bearing only one 2-cent redemption stamp, and good only when it carried 52 2-cent stamps, quickly would lead to disaster. It simply cannot be done. The claim that it can be done reveals the unsoundness of the whole proposition and the inexperience and recklessness of those who back it.*

It is possible that the transparent cynicism of this strategem backfired on the Ham and Eggs movement, for on election day the measure did not carry a single county and lost in the state by al-

---

* Long Beach *Press-Telegram*, Oct. 21, 1939. In fairness to the Ham and Eggers it should be said that under this proposal warrants would be cashed for one dollar only if they had at least six two-cent stamps. Warrants circulated for 30 days would have four stamps, and the new proposal provided that in order to be redeemed they would have to be stamped two additional weeks in advance. Thus the Ham and Eggers would give a person a dollar not for two cents but for twelve—still quite a bargain.

most one million votes. The final count was 1,933,557 to 993,204.[107]
For all practical purposes, Ham and Eggs was finished in California.

Yet the Ham and Eggers were far from ready to call it quits.
They had announced before the election that they would continue
their campaign, and Willis Allen declared in his first public statement after the election, "Our fight must go on. . . . It will go on."[108]
Asserting that the near-million electors who had voted with them
("A Million Who Can't Be Scared") gave them a balance of power
in California, the leaders proposed to place still another Ham and
Eggs initiative on the ballot and to start a move to recall Governor Olson.[109]

The recall campaign began immediately. Declaring Olson had
forgotten his "friends" in the Ham and Eggs movement and had
"actively campaigned on behalf of the bankers and monopolies,"
the Ham and Eggs leaders concluded, "Governor Olson has demonstrated . . . that not only is he incapable of solving the problems
now facing the state, he is incapable of allowing these problems
to be solved by others.[110] They took the Governor sharply to task
for suddenly advocating higher old-age pensions after the election
and declared, probably correctly, that the Governor's new position
was merely an attempt to regain the support of the old people
whom he had alienated by his opposition to Ham and Eggs.[111] The
leaders also struck a sensitive nerve when they predicted accur-
ately that the proposal to increase pensions would be defeated by
the "reactionary" legislature, and they especially embarrassed
Olson by publicizing the fact that some of his closest associates
were against the measure.[112] Finally, when the Ham and Eggers
decided to merge their recall movement with an identical movement led by a more conservative group, it began to appear as
though their campaign might be successful.[113]

The new RLPA initiative campaign was also inaugurated with
the usual blare and bounce. Early in December the Ham and Eggs
editors announced the coming of a "progressive educational campaign" for the purpose of "selling our revised amendment to the
voters," and subsequently they informed their readers that the
new amendment would be a streamlined version of the previous
one, retaining its basic features and eliminating its objectionable
aspects.[114] After further ballyhoo, the leaders released the text of

this new "miracle." Its main provisions were: the payment of pensions in stamp scrip of $20 a week, rather than $30, to all unemployed persons who were 50 or over; the creation of a state-owned bank capitalized at $20 million; the replacement of all existing state taxes by a 3 per cent gross income tax (churches, schools, and charitable institutions were to be exempt); and the election of a a three-man board one of whose members would again be either Roy Owens or Will Kindig, to administer the act.[115] Once again California seemed destined to be the scene of a bizarre Ham and Eggs political campaign.

This new movement was not long in finding opponents, and one of the most effective proved once more to be Governor Olson himself. Emerging at last as a full-fledged opponent of Ham and Eggs, he began his counterattack by trying to persuade the public, and perhaps himself, that he had always taken that position. Early in December 1939 he made a ringing, though not very convincing, disavowal of the authorship of the telegrams in which he had endorsed Ham and Eggs in the 1938 primary.* He then proceeded to oppose the Ham and Eggers in both their initiative and their recall movement. In so doing he gained the support of some of the more conservative elements that had previously opposed him. One formerly anti-Olson newspaper, for example, bitterly denounced the Ham and Eggs recall campaign:

The entire proposition STINKS.

It STINKS just as badly, if not worse, than the CARRION leadership of the Ham and Eggs movement.

STINK is not a pleasant word. It means "giving forth a foul aroma." Used as an adjective, carrion means the "aroma from dead flesh."

---

* On December 3, 1939, Olson declared that the two telegrams "were not written by me nor sent in the form desired by me," but had been written and sent by some "other person"—probably a reference to Nathan T. Porter. Furthermore, the Governor said that the 1938 Ham and Eggs measure "would have done irreparable harm, but would have lasted only a few months and we could have recovered from it," whereas the 1939 measure "would have worked permanent and irreparable damage." Los Angeles *Times*, Dec. 4, 1939. The *Times* inquired the next day why the Governor had not opposed the 1938 measure and why he had called an election for it if he thought it would be so harmful. And why had he waited two years to repudiate the telegrams if he had neither written nor sent them? These were telling points to which Olson never responded. Porter, for his part, castigated the Governor for what seemed to be transparent dishonesty and declared that Olson had both written and signed the telegrams in question. *National Ham and Eggs*, Dec. 9, Dec. 23, 1939.

California would be well off if it could get to work on a sound old-age program, improving what we have already created, and should bury this foul dead flesh which has been exposed for two long years to the air of an otherwise enlightened state.[116]

The Ham and Eggs movement, by its refusal to die after two election defeats, produced a sense of frustration and outrage among its opponents that unified them as never before.

At the same time, the unity of the RLPA was breaking. Several of the leaders, the most important of them being Charles M. Hawks, had long resented the high-handed tactics of the Allens, and they apparently disagreed with the decision to launch the recall drive.[117] According to the remaining leaders, these dissidents then entered into a conspiracy with Olson's henchmen to destroy the recall drive by a premature filing of recall petitions, thereby limiting the time remaining to secure the needed number of signatures to 40 days.[118] Although the defectors were ejected from the organization and the rank-and-file members supposedly supported the remaining leadership, the recall movement lapsed, especially after a Ham and Eggs slate in the presidential primary of 1940 was disastrously defeated by the pro-Roosevelt slate, headed by Governor Olson.[119]

The new Ham and Eggs initiative campaign also declined rapidly in the summer of 1940. The petition drive had been inaugurated in February with the slogan "$30 a Week for Life—$20 Now" and the usual high-powered propaganda assuring the public that the measure would easily qualify for a place on the ballot.[120] Some groups were so fearful that it would qualify and were so utterly weary with the continual threat of Ham and Eggs elections that they began to advocate reform of the initiative laws to prohibit defeated measures from reappearing on the ballot until a certain period of time had elapsed.[121] As it turned out, no such tactic was needed, for the Ham and Eggs measure failed to win enough signatures to qualify on the 1940 ballot. Still unwilling to give up, the leaders claimed that they had been robbed in the counting and validation of these signatures, but their plea was dismissed by the court.[122]

Deprived of an immediately impending ballot measure to sustain the interest of the voters, the RLPA quickly drifted into apathy. The leaders feebly participated in the 1940 primaries by endorsing four congressional candidates, all of whom lost spectacularly, and they tried to arouse new enthusiasm after the election by inaugurating a so-called square-deal campaign.[123] This innocuous gesture was a grab bag of reform proposals solicited from the membership, for the ostensible purpose of producing a new initiative measure. Eventually some 39 "breath-taking proposals" were put forth, ranging from the abolition of parking meters and the regulation of football-ticket sales to the establishment of a unicameral legislature and the abolition of the state bar association.[124] Suffice it to say that this program had nothing to do with the old-age pension movement, and nothing whatever came of it. It was obviously a desperate attempt to sustain enthusiasm and to keep up financial contributions until a new election appeal could be made.

The attempt failed. Despite urgent pleas for financial pledges to "keep the doors open," revenues declined sharply in 1940, Ham and Eggs meetings and other activities decreased in number, and the party newspaper dwindled in size.[125] The organization's only hope was to stay alive until 1942, when the initiative amendment that had failed to qualify in 1940 would supposedly be put to a vote. The Ham and Eggers had continued to gather signatures after the filing deadline in 1940 and soon claimed that they had succeeded in qualifying the measure for the 1942 election. But in October 1940 the Secretary of State delivered a coup de grace to the movement when he disqualified some 14,000 of the petition signatures, thereby eliminating the measure from the 1942 ballot.[126] Although Willis Allen shouted defiance at the "Sacramento Hitlers" who had thus defeated him and declared that the decision would not "go unchallenged," it was a futile gesture, for at long last the Ham and Eggs movement was finished.

7

Governor Olson's New Deal

WHEN Culbert L. Olson won election to the governorship in 1938 on a pledge to "bring the New Deal to California," there were many besides himself who thought he would be able to do it. After all, he seemed to have brought the state at last into line with the "Roosevelt revolution," and his election reflected the growing strength of the California Democratic Party. The Democrats had gained control of the state Assembly in 1936 and had made great inroads into the Republican majority in the Senate, and by 1938 the party was numerically superior to the Republican Party in registered voters.[1] Furthermore, in electing Olson, an avowed New Dealer with a clear-cut liberal-EPIC record in the state legislature,[2] the voters had, so it seemed to him, given him a clear mandate to secure the enactment of the far-reaching liberal program he had advocated in his campaign. With such assurances of widespread political support, Culbert Olson seemed confident that California was to have a new birth of progressivism and that he had been chosen to bring it about.

These hopes, however, were unalloyed illusions. The New Deal tide in 1938 was receding rather than advancing in California, as in the nation at large, and the Republicans were beginning to regain legislative strength on both fronts.[3] In 1939, when Governor Olson submitted his first New Deal program to the legislature, he had a slim majority of eight Democratic seats in the Assembly, and in the Senate he was in the minority by five.[4] Furthermore, the Democratic legislators were hardly likely to respond positively to the leadership of the Governor, or for that matter, anyone else. Reflecting the typical maverick tendencies of California's weak party system, the Democrats were even more undisciplined than the Republicans,[5] and many Democrats in the legislature turned out to be more conservative as well. Their opposition to Olson's liberalism was foreshadowed when only four Senate Democrats voted to give the liberal Lieutenant Governor Ellis Patterson a voice in appointing senatorial committees. The Assembly did choose an Olsonite, Paul Peek, as Speaker, but only after considerable disapproval of him was expressed by conservatives in the Democratic ranks.[6]

Apparently oblivious to this opposition, Olson submitted to the legislature a detailed program of reform that was made to order for arousing opposition in conservative circles. This program aimed to increase social services mainly by expanding the budgets of state welfare and regulatory agencies and state institutions, and it proposed to finance the increased expenditures (the proposed budget amounted to $557 million) by imposing higher taxes on those most able to pay.[7] It was, in short, a model of progressive reform that could be passed only in a state where special interest lobbies were weak, where public sentiment for reform was strong, where liberal legislators were dominant and able, and where party discipline held. Since in California none of these conditions prevailed, Culbert Olson was headed for frustration and defeat.

While the legislature was cutting his program to pieces, the Governor had a number of other misfortunes that further weakened his leadership. Early in January 1939 he suffered a nervous and physical collapse and was confined to his bed for several weeks.[8] Because of this he lost touch with political developments at the very time when his opponents were combining to defeat his program. Early in April he suffered another shock when his wife died suddenly.[9] In the meantime he had incurred the enmity of many of the state's more fanatic conservatives by pardoning labor martyr Thomas Mooney, the "American Dreyfus," who had languished in prison since 1916. For this act of simple justice he was deluged with angry messages accusing him of committing a crime against the state; one even threatened ominously that he would "surely pay the toll."[10]

The toll Olson paid was the destruction of his legislative program. By the end of the 1939 session a conservative coalition of Republicans and Democrats, shouting the old slogan "No New

Taxes," reduced the Governor's budget by $90 million, curtailed social services, emasculated his relief program, and defeated every one of his revenue proposals except the relatively insignificant gift tax.[11] This legislative debacle was typical of the political shambles that characterized most of Governor Olson's administration.

In these inauspicious circumstances, the older age groups at first were also largely frustrated in their attempts to secure favorable legislation. And here a curious fact came to light. Sponsors of proposals to liberalize the Old-Age Security Act soon found that they could expect opposition not only from economizers in the legislature but from the Governor himself. He had advocated "state aid for the aged to the limit that public finances [would] permit" in his campaign for the governorship in 1938; but when he repeated this statement in his inaugural address, he added an important qualification. "That limit," he said, "may for a time, at least, be very nearly reached." Although he admitted that "the amount of the pension is too low and the age limit too high," Olson declared correctly that the California pension of $35 a month, "however inadequate, is more liberal than that paid by any other state." Furthermore, to raise the pension, he argued, would not only strain the state's finances seriously but would bring old people from other states flocking into California to take advantage of its generosity. The only solution to the problem, Olson asserted, was a uniform national old-age pension system financed entirely by the federal government.[12] Thus early in his administration Governor Olson took an unsympathetic stand on increased old-age pensions, and afterward he was never able to convince most of the old people that he was their friend.

Why did Olson take this stand? Apparently he had concluded, and perhaps with considerable justification, that persons drawing old-age benefits were, despite the inadequacy of their pensions, better cared for than other unfortunates, such as the unemployed and their families; and the state, he seemed to think, simply could not at that time afford to do more than attempt to alleviate the distress of those who suffered most acutely from the Depression. Since he felt the aged did not fall into that category, they would have to be content for the time being with the meager benefits of the Old-Age Security Act, unless the federal government could be persuaded to come to their aid.[13]

The economic justification of this position, however, was offset by the political ineptitude with which the Governor presented it. The call for federal aid was seemingly an empty gesture, and Olson's revival of the bogey of an army of aged paupers waiting to descend on the state contributed to the stereotype of the older age groups as hobos and spongers. In the long run, Olson's tactless rebuff of the old-age pensioners largely cost him their support at a time when he could not afford to lose support from any quarter. Moreover, his attitude doubtless contributed heavily to the burgeoning strength of the Ham and Eggs movement. Thus Olson's estrangement from the older age groups contributed to the frustration of both, and to the success of their common enemies.

The legislative session of 1939 provides a good example of the way the Governor and the pension movement canceled each other out. While the legislature was making hash out of Olson's social service, relief, and tax programs without any strong protests from the pension movement, Olson acquiesced completely in the legislature's defeat of attempts to raise monthly old-age pensions to $50 or more.[14] Furthermore, when the legislature passed a measure appropriating $6.7 million from the state treasury to help counties defray the cost of old-age pensions, Olson vetoed the measure. Although many old people could probably see no excuse for Olson's action, his reasoning was logical enough: the state had no funds for such an appropriation because the legislature had defeated his revenue proposals.[15]

Seemingly far less defensible was Olson's veto of a bill to grant pensions to inmates of private charitable institutions to help them pay the fees for staying there.[16] The Governor gave no reason for this veto, although again the obstacle was probably a financial one. The veto meant, however, that if an aged inmate of such an institution was no longer able to pay his fees, he would have to leave the institution and either attempt to live on a pension or enter a county hospital. It is difficult to believe that Olson really thought the state's financial condition precluded the passage of this relatively minor economic measure, especially when vetoing the bill was likely to arouse the political displeasure of the aged. If the veto was an attempt to discredit the legislature, it was largely unsuccessful, and in the end the Governor probably discredited no one as much as himself.

The older age groups did, however, score some successes in the 1939 session. They secured the passage of two memorials to Congress, one calling for a national old-age pension system and the other requesting that the federal pension grant be doubled.[17] They also induced the legislature to lengthen from 30 days to 60 days the time a pensioner could stay in a public hospital for temporary medical care, and to exempt a responsible relative from contributing to a pensioner's support if the relative had not filed a state income tax return.[18] This latter provision greatly simplified the procedure for determining whether or not relatives should be held responsible and probably lessened considerably the ill feeling that was often created between a pensioner and his family by the relative-responsibility clause.

The older age groups also secured enactments to deal with a perennial grievance, the lien provision of the Old-Age Security Act. The 1939 legislature passed a law giving the counties discretionary authority to release liens and encumbrances on pensioners' property, and in case this law was declared unconstitutional, as had happened in 1938, the legislature also passed a proposed constitutional amendment specifically repealing all such liens.[19] Thus a clear-cut victory seemed to have been won.

However, there was a catch to the lien law of 1939. While it authorized each county to release liens on pensioners' property, it also allowed the county to require a pensioner to make an agreement not to transfer or encumber his property without permission, on pain of forfeiting his pension. And it also gave the county the general right of an unsecured creditor against the recipient's estate, including the right to claim reimbursement after his death for the amount of aid granted.[20] In short, the legislature seemed to be taking away with one hand what it granted with the other. The pensioners and applicants saw no real difference between a lien provision and an unsecured creditor clause, since both clouded the titles to their property and undermined their cherished right to bequeath their property to their heirs, and provisions against transferring or encumbering property seemed even more galling.[21] Indeed, the new provision proved so odious to pensioners that within the following year some 4,000 of them chose to give up their pensions altogether rather than execute such agreements; for the first time in the history of the Old-Age Security Act the number of pensioners decreased.[22] Thus to the dismay of the old people, another victory had turned to ashes.

By the end of the 1939 session Governor Olson's political position was weak. He had proved inept in handling the legislature, and he had forfeited the support of large segments of the older age groups. The conservative forces had demonstrated great strength, and radical movements like Ham and Eggs seemed to hold a powerful attraction for the disillusioned and the dissatisfied.[23] Olson resolved to do better in the future.

The Governor had a great deal of political fencemending to do, especially among the older age groups. He had alienated the old people not only by his unsympathetic attitude toward their legislative proposals but by his militant opposition to the Ham and Eggs amendment. For this reason, within a week after the Ham and Eggs election of 1939, Olson announced his sponsorship of what came to be called the Sixty-Sixty movement. This movement's program was to memorialize Congress to lower the minimum age for old-age pensioners under the Social Security Act to 60 and to raise the maximum pension to $60 a month. The plan also called for full federal financing of the program, but Olson declared that until Congress acted he would request the California legislature to at least make a start on the program by lowering the minimum age to 60.[24] Shortly afterward Lieutenant Governor Ellis Patterson strongly endorsed the Sixty-Sixty plan by calling a special meeting of northern California legislators and urging them to support the proposal.[25] Patterson's action may have gained Olson some support among the aged, since Patterson, it will be remembered, had actively supported the Ham and Eggs scheme.

But the Sixty-Sixty plan reaped a harvest of abuse from other quarters. Conservatives declared, as usual, that the program would be too costly and would attract swarms of aged indigents into the state.[26] Others, who had come to hate Olson for various liberal measures he had advocated, called him radical and irresponsible.*
But the Governor, seemingly undeterred by the powerful opposi-

* Among the Governor's more vocal critics at this time were some labor unions, which feared his production-for-use proposals; business and political conservatives, who were enraged by his tax proposals; and the notoriously conservative Associated Farmers, who hated Olson for his "partisan support of the LaFollette committee's civil liberties investigation of agricultural labor conditions in California." Pasadena *Star-News*, Dec. 12, 1939.

tion being organized against him, announced that he was calling a special session of the legislature early in 1940 and would submit to it a legislative reform program almost as extensive as the one that had been so soundly defeated in the previous session. Despite the fact that his enemies were stronger than before and he was politically weaker, Olson asked the special session for liberalized old-age pensions, more relief funds, new taxes, the creation of a state housing authority, the reorganization of certain government departments, and a public power program to be financed by a revenue bond issue. "Governor Olson has put everything but the kitchen sink into his agenda," fulminated one irate newspaper editor.[27] In view of the mounting cries for economy at Sacramento, Olson's prospects for realizing his varied goals in the special session of 1940 seemed poor at best.

The debacle began immediately. Before the session was over the Governor had been subjected to one of the most humiliating series of defeats in the history of California politics. On the first day of the session, a group of conservative Democrats in the Assembly joined forces with the Republicans to unseat Paul Peek as Speaker and elect in his stead an outspoken anti-Olson Democrat named Gordon Garland.[28] Garland symbolically severed relations with the Governor when he tore out the telephone connection that supposedly linked the Speaker's desk with the Governor's office and announced that he intended to reverse "the increasing trend toward collectivism."[29] Seizing on Olson's request for a modest relief appropriation, the legislature charged that the State Relief Administration was dominated by Communists and reduced the appropriation to a fraction of Olson's request, even though unemployment had been rising rapidly during the winter of 1939–40, bringing acute distress to jobless families.[30] Then, to Olson's great embarrassment, the Sacramento *Bee* made the sensational disclosure that one of Olson's aides had placed a hidden dictograph in Speaker Garland's hotel room. Amid charges that the Governor was not only a radical but an unscrupulous dictator, the legislature went on to defeat almost every one of his major proposals and to make a shambles of his New Deal program once more.[31]

Not surprisingly, the proposal to liberalize old-age pensions was one of the casualties of this reaction. True to his word, Olson had called for a reduction of the pension age to 60, but when an Assembly bill to this effect was introduced, it was quickly tabled and never revived.[32] Other bills to increase the state funds available for old-age pensions also failed to pass.[33] Furthermore, the older age groups suffered two setbacks in 1940, when the California Attorney General ruled that income pensioners derived from employer annuity plans and from compensation for industrial accidents must be deducted from old-age pension checks.[34] Although both of these rulings were doubtless warranted, they probably made old people feel more antagonistic than ever about bureaucratic technicalities that prevented them from getting what they thought was their due.*

More important to the pensioners, however, was their drive to repeal the previous year's provision requiring a pensioner to agree not to transfer or encumber his property without permission from the county. And here the older age groups, despite the prevailing conservatism of the times, scored a clear victory. The fight over this provision, which will be called here simply the nonencumbrance provision, was one of the rare occasions when the Townsend organization exerted effective leadership in California. In the summer of 1939 the Townsendites attacked the provision and began to pressure county boards to ignore it.[35] This seemed a feasible approach, especially after Attorney General Earl Warren ruled that that the nonencumbrance provision could be applied at the discretion of the counties.[36] The Los Angeles County Board accordingly decided to disregard the provision after being petitioned to do so by a delegation of Townsendites, but the supervisors of Alameda County turned down the request of a similar delegation.[37]

A much greater setback occurred in December 1939. The state Department of Social Welfare ruled that despite the discretionary language of the law, all counties must apply the nonencumbrance provision in order to meet the federal Social Security Act requirement that a pension system be administered uniformly throughout the state. Failure to do so, it was argued, would make the state

---

* Also at about this time a California judge denied the naturalization petition of an aged applicant on the ground that his only motive in seeking citizenship was to be eligible for a pension, and the Sacramento County Board of Supervisors confiscated $600 of a total of $1,100 a pensioner had saved from his old-age pension checks on the ground that the law allowed a pensioner to have only $500 in personal property. Los Angeles *Times*, Dec. 19, 1940; Sacramento *Bee*, May 15, May 21, 1940.

ineligible to receive federal Social Security grants for old-age pensions.[38] Not surprisingly, this ruling was met by a storm of opposition. Senator Ralph Swing of San Bernardino County threatened court action against county officials who enforced it, and the Los Angeles County supervisors voted to disregard it.[39] But when the Department of Social Welfare decided to withhold the state's share of old-age pension funds from Los Angeles County until it complied with the ruling, the county capitulated over the strenuous objections of the Townsendites.[40] When similar decisions were made in San Francisco and Sonoma counties, it became obvious that the only way to fight the nonencumbrance provision was to induce the legislature to repeal it.*

This proved to be amazingly easy. On the first day of the special session of 1940, Governor Olson asked that the unpopular provision be repealed; within two days a bill repealing it was introduced in the state Senate, and a week later the bill passed unanimously.[41] This bill, however, contained an amendment depriving the state Department of Social Welfare of the power to withhold state pension funds from a county that violated the department's rules (as had just been done in Los Angeles County). When the Assembly was advised by the federal Social Security director that this amendment would in effect transfer the control of aged welfare from the state to the counties and hence fall afoul of the federal uniformity rule, the Assembly refused to pass the bill.[42] But in the meantime another bill repealing the nonencumbrance provision had been introduced, and with widespread support from the aged, it passed both houses in a mere two weeks with but one dissenting vote.[43] Olson signed the measure, while priding himself on having called for its adoption. Later he could point to it as one of the few enlightened enactments of that otherwise disastrous session.[44]

Still the opponents of the nonencumbrance provision were not

---

* San Francisco *Chronicle*, Jan. 30, 1940; Santa Rosa *Press-Democrat*, Jan. 24, 1940. The Sonoma County grand jury passed a resolution favoring the retention of the nonencumbrance provision on the grounds that it was a legitimate device to prevent children who had refused to support their parents from acquiring their parents' property after their deaths and to enable the county to recover some of what it had spent for pensions. *Ibid.* Reasonable as this argument might have seemed, it failed to recognize the emotional consequences of undermining a pensioner's property rights. Other counties had by this time spoken out in favor of repealing the nonencumbrance provision. *Ibid.*

satisfied. There remained the possibility that the state Supreme Court would declare the repeal measure unconstitutional, as it had the lien repeal act two years before. As we have seen, the 1939 legislature had responded to the Supreme Court's decision by placing a constitutional amendment before the voters to legalize the lien repeal, but this amendment did not apply specifically to the nonencumbrance provision. For this reason a demand arose for a second constitutional amendment to release all pensioners from nonencumbrance agreements they had made. Accordingly, the legislature unanimously passed a constitutional amendment to repeal the provision in even less time than it had taken to pass the bill repealing the lien provision, and it also rammed through a special enabling act to put this proposition in the first place on the ballot in the 1940 election.[45] Thus the lien repeal amendment became known as Proposition Two, and the nonencumbrance repeal amendment, which also included a lien repeal just to be on the safe side, became Proposition One.[46]

A strenuous campaign was waged over the two amendments.[47] The Townsendites tried to capitalize on the enthusiasm for liberalizing the Old-Age Security Act by proposing a third constitutional amendment much more sweeping in nature than propositions One and Two, and although their initiative failed to qualify for a place on the ballot, their agitation probably helped generate support for the other two proposals.[48] A month before the election the California Supreme Court gave great encouragement to the pension leaders when in the case of *Alameda v. Janssen* it upheld the discretionary authority of the counties to release liens on pensioners' property, thereby reversing its decision of two years before.[49] On November 5, 1940, the voters approved both propositions by margins of more than a half-million votes, and the quarrels over liens and nonencumbrance agreements were finally eliminated from old-age politics in California.[50]

This accomplishment must be rated a considerable triumph for the older age groups. In the face of a conservative reaction that had shattered the Governor's New Deal program, the pension leaders were able to win over both the legislature and the electorate. It is likely, of course, that neither the legislature nor the voters considered the lien and nonencumbrance issues of major importance, since they had small economic significance. To the aged, however, these issues were vital, because if they did not affect a pensioner's income, they did affect his status. And in many cases status probably seemed more important.

Furthermore, by 1940 the California pensioner could find some economic blessings to count. Paying an average pension of $38 a month, California led all the other states in size of individual grants.[51] Although pension spokesmen were prone to decry the "niggardliness" of the California taxpayer, it is worth noting that the average tax paid by real property owners toward old-age pensions rose from one cent per $100 at the beginning of the 1930's to 24 cents per $100 at the decade's close.[52] By 1940 the average annual cost of old-age pensions in California for each employed worker was $25.74, whereas the average cost in the nation at large was only $10.52.[53] The per capita costs of old-age pensions in California and the United States at the beginning of 1940 were $8.34 and $3.33 respectively.[54] On the other side, it must be said that the proportion of California's 65-and-over population receiving pensions was only 25 per cent, not appreciably higher than the national average and considerably lower than the proportion in at least a dozen states. Still, in 1940 California spent more for old-age pensions ($64,930,770) and had more old-age pensioners (150,576) than any other state.[55] Such achievements were no small matter to the older age groups.

If the pension movement had made significant progress during Olson's administration, little of that progress can be credited to Olson himself. So far as the old people were concerned, the Governor's New Deal had been a failure, and they probably contributed heavily to his defeat at the polls in 1942. In his stead, Californians elected Earl Warren, who had campaigned loudly for improving the old-age pension system.[56] The pension movement's ability to survive the resurgence of conservatism during the Olson administration is an indication that by 1940 the older age groups had taken a firm hold in California politics. They had transformed themselves from a disorganized and heterogeneous group whose problems were ignored by the rest of the community into a self-conscious and highly vocal interest group. In short, they had secured a considerable amount of political power by 1940, and they have wielded it with authority and effectiveness ever since.

8

The Continuing Crusade
1940–69

OWING TO the older age groups' continued political activity since 1940, California probably still has the most comprehensive aged welfare program in the country.[1] A number of general circumstances have contributed to their success: the momentum of public support engendered during the 1930's on both the state and national levels; the return of prosperity during and after the war; and the resurgence of political progressivism in California, beginning with Governor Warren's administration and reaching new heights during Governor Brown's. Perhaps more fundamental, the problems of the aged have proved persistent, despite the gains made in the 1930's, and aged Californians have proved equally persistent in their determination to solve them.[2]

The older age groups' most important secret of success, however, is that they have become better organized and have turned increasingly to the tactics of pressure politics. To be sure, the earlier organizations were fading after 1940, and although a crackpot medley of new groups emerged under the leadership of former Ham and Eggers and the like, they were, with one singular exception, transitory and unimportant.[3] The exception was an organization led by George McLain, a powerful figure who quickly came to dominate organized pension politics in California.

McLain was perfectly suited to his role. A native Californian with a somewhat genteel background, he saw at first hand the sufferings of the elderly during the Great Depression, when his father, whose business had been ruined, was forced to submit to the humiliations of trying to secure a pension under the Old-Age Security Act.[4] McLain's sense of indignation took him first into feeble and futile attempts to win political office and then into the Ham and Eggs movement. There he apparently learned the value of political propaganda and organization, as well as the folly of staking everything on sweeping utopian schemes to the exclusion of piecemeal reform.

In 1940 McLain left the Ham and Eggs organization, apparently in an unfriendly mood, and took some other angry defectors with him. Shortly thereafter he attached himself to the newly organized American Citizens' Pension Association, a group he soon supplanted with one of his own.[5] Although McLain's organization has had many names—it has been known successively as the Old-Age Payment Campaign Committee, the Citizens' Committee for Old-Age Pensions, the California Institute of Social Welfare, and the California League of Senior Citizens (CLSC)—McLain's control of it remained undiminished until his death in July 1965.[6] Since then the organization has remained largely intact, with McLain's long-time associate Myrtle Williams serving as chairman, and his son George McLain, Jr., as secretary-treasurer.

McLain was never reluctant to use the political power he derived from the support of the older age groups, and he became both widely revered and fiercely hated as a consequence. He sprang into prominence after the election of 1948, when to everyone's surprise he secured the passage of a constitutional amendment that greatly liberalized the provisions of the Old-Age Security Act and transferred the administration of the act entirely from the counties to a new state agency under the direction of his chief lieutenant, Myrtle Williams.[7] Although this measure was repealed the following year and McLain never won another election,[8] his popularity was not diminished. In the 1960 presidential primary election he showed his political muscle by winning an astounding 646,387 votes, almost half as many as the favorite-son candidate, Governor Edmund G. Brown.[9]

Although during the 1960 presidential primary campaign McLain accused Brown of neglecting the older age groups, the two later became political allies. In 1962 McLain strongly backed Brown's bid for reelection against Richard Nixon, who was accused of being hostile toward aged welfare legislation.[10] In return Brown not only helped secure the passage of some of McLain's legislative proposals and publicly praised his efforts on behalf of the aged, but also appointed him to the Citizens Advisory Committee on Aging and gave him other forms of recognition that enhanced his status.[11]

It is not difficult to catalog the more questionable features of McLain's "establishment," and a number of able scholars have done so.[12] In particular, the partisan tone of his propaganda casts discredit on his organization. His constant exploitation of the themes of society's persecution and alienation of the aged tended to reinforce the very feeling of alienation he purported to combat, so that his followers were encouraged to depend on him rather than on society at large to help them solve their problems. His absolute control of the organization made them even more dependent on him. His incessant demands for money to aid the "cause" not only sounded suspicious to the outside observer but aroused guilt feelings among the generally indigent rank and file, who he often complained had let him down. And his willingness to use the organization as a political machine in his attempts to gain political office raised doubts about the sincerity of his motives.

There is much to be said, however, in McLain's defense. If he exploited the alienation theme, he did not invent it. For that matter, the alienation of the aged amounted to a social fact of life, and any political solution to the problem would inevitably mean at least some political exploitation of it. If McLain's propaganda was partisan, it was probably no more so than that of his most vehement opponents, who castigated him as a mere "promoter" and implied that the older age groups had no legitimate grievances whatever. The undemocratic structure of the organization seemingly reflected not only McLain's elitist tastes but also the utter lack of leadership talents among the rank and file. His repeated appeals for funds were no doubt necessitated by the high cost of operating a large political organization, and there is no evidence that McLain ever used these funds for any illegitimate purpose. The fact that McLain was politically ambitious is not in itself a mark against him; his own argument that he could be more effective if he held political office was at least a plausible explanation.

McLain's strongest defense, however, is his unremitting effort to secure old-age legislation in Sacramento. Unlike the Townsendites, the Ham and Eggers, and other groups, he largely abjured sweeping panaceas. He early made his peace with the Old-Age Security Act and devoted himself to bringing about legislative improvements in it. Since 1941 first McLain and then his successors have operated a so-called old-folks' lobby, which functions vigorously at every session of the California legislature. Although the lobby has probably been less influential than McLain sometimes claimed, it has clearly played an important role in the continuing liberalization of the aged welfare program in California during the last thirty years.[13]

What gains have the older age groups made? The most basic is perhaps the steady increase in the number of persons who draw a state or federal old-age pension, or both. Whereas some 151,000 Californians were drawing state pensions in December 1941, nearly 275,000 were drawing them ten years later.[14] Although a decline set in between 1952 and 1966, successive liberalizations of the law reversed the trend, and by mid-1969 some 301,000 aged Californians were drawing pensions under the Old-Age Security Act.[15]

The decline in the number of pensioners in the 1950's and early 1960's, furthermore, was not due to any reaction against the older age groups. Instead it was entirely due to the increased coverage of California's aged by federal Old-Age and Survivors Insurance (OASI) under the Social Security Act. In fact, California and federal welfare officials specifically intended that the state pension system should serve as a transition measure until the federal system covered all the elderly.[16] Although this goal is far from realized as yet, the successive liberalizations of the Social Security Act in 1950, 1952, 1954, 1956, 1958, 1960, 1961, 1965, 1967, and 1969 have indeed shifted the bulk of the burden for old-age welfare in California from the state to the federal government.[17] Whereas some 30 per cent of California's 65-and-over population were drawing state pensions at the end of 1950, less than 20 per cent were drawing them by the end of 1960. And at the same time the percentage of the state's aged population drawing federal pensions under OASI increased from about 27 per cent to almost 70 per cent.[18] Thus a large majority of California's aged population is at least partly dependent on the state or federal government, or both, for its livelihood. If the percentage of state pensioners has decreased, however, the cost of pensions has not. The fact that total old-age pension expenditures in California increased from $68 million in fiscal 1940–41 to $223 million in fiscal 1950–51, and to $375 million in fiscal 1968–69, is a striking demonstration of the abiding influence of the older age groups in California politics.[19]

Pension costs have increased, of course, because the legislature has repeatedly liberalized the pension law. In 1941 the state inaugurated a "special needs" policy whereby a person whose income was too high to qualify him for a pension could secure a pension anyway if he had special needs, such as medical care, whose cost would otherwise overburden him.[20] This policy made many more persons eligible for pensions and kept the rolls large. In addition, during the Warren and Knight administrations the legislature repeatedly increased the maximum grant, from $40 a month in 1940 to $50 in 1943, $60 in 1947, $65 in 1948, $75 in 1949, $80 in 1952, $85 in 1955, and $89 in 1956.[21] In 1957 the legislature enlarged on the special-needs provision by awarding an additional $16 a month above the maximum grant to pensioners who had special needs but little or no outside income with which to meet them.[22] This change raised the maximum regular and special-needs pensions to $89 and $105 respectively, and these figures have also been repeatedly increased—to $90 and $106 in 1958, $95 and $115 in 1959, and $101 and $166 in 1961. In 1961 a cost-of-living adjustment system was initiated, and as a result the current minimum and maximum benefits are respectively $129 and $194.[23] To be sure, not everyone drew pensions this size, but the average monthly pension did increase from $36.51 in December 1941 to $66.59 in December 1951, $78.34 in December 1961, and $103.62 in July 1969.[24] Such increases, whether or not they could be regarded as generous, have helped to make old-age pension expenditures one of the major items in the state's budget.*

Not only has the legislature raised pensions; it has also made more people eligible to draw them. The property qualifications

---

* It is well to remember that approximately one-half the cost of these old-age pension payments was and is borne by the federal government. Nevertheless, California must be credited with supporting this program to a much higher degree than the rest of the nation. In 1940 the average cost of state old-age pensions to each employed worker in the United States was $10.52, whereas in California it was $25.74; in 1950 the respective figures were $25.99 and $58.30. Floyd A. Bond et al., *Our Needy Aged: A California Study of a National Problem* (New York, 1954), inside front cover and pp. 218–48. I have been unable to find similar statistics for 1960 and after.

have been successively liberalized, both by upward revisions of special-needs estimates and by outright increases in the amounts of personal and real property a pensioner may own.[25] Beginning in 1943 the controversial relative-responsibility clause was successively amended in favor of the pensioners and their children, and today the clause is practically inapplicable in the vast majority of cases. No doubt this victory has brought considerable emotional satisfaction to the elderly.[26] The citizenship requirement was first modified in favor of Japanese-Americans and then eliminated altogether.[27] And a host of amendments streamlined the administration of the Old-Age Security Act, relieving pensioners of much of the official harassment and red tape they had formerly complained of.[28] Such reforms clearly demonstrate the legislature's sustained sensitivity to the economic problems of the older age groups.

Nor was the legislature sensitive only to the economic problems of the aged. Perhaps the greatest single achievement of California's old-age pension movement during the past two decades has been to increase public awareness of the social and psychological problems that often cause the aged more profound distress than mere economic considerations. The public has begun to accept the idea that the problems of the aged may call for a fundamental reordering of the relationship between the older age groups and the rest of society. "During this biennium," an official statement read in 1950,

there has been a slowly growing appreciation of the fact that old people require more than economic security in order to live a normal life. There is greater recognition that any person, regardless of age, must continue to be a functioning and integral part of his community. He has the need to continue in his own behalf and in the interests of society as long as he is able to do so. To retire to a purposeless and enforced leisure is to die mentally, spiritually, and physically. Hence, it becomes a matter of vital importance to encourage him to use his capacities for his own support as well as to contribute to the life of those around him.[29]

California political leaders have been instrumental at least in articulating and publicizing these new viewpoints. In 1957 the Department of Social Welfare officially restated its policy on old-age security by declaring the necessity not only of increasing individual incomes but of helping old people "retain their feelings of value as persons and their individual independence."[30] In 1962 another state agency issued an attractive brochure entitled "California Cares about Its Elder Citizens," which pointed out the far-reaching problems of the aged and showed how the state was attempting to deal with them.[31] At about the same time the state legislature passed a resolution designating May 1962 Senior Citizens Month. The resolution urged California communities to "stress the importance of the contribution to the welfare and well-being of the entire community which can be made by the senior citizens," and to make their communities "places where the senior citizen can live out his years in dignity, self-respect, usefulness, and good citizenship."[32] Governor Brown, in his proclamation making Senior Citizens Month official, also emphasized the "talent, wisdom, and experience of California's older people" and praised the efforts of various old-age organizations to make use of their skills.[33] In various public addresses to old-age organizations, Brown not only reiterated these themes but pointed out the many steps taken by his administration on behalf of the aged.[34]

Governor Brown was obviously proud of his administration's record. One significant advance was to stimulate grass-roots interest in the problems of the aged by promoting various community projects. The Department of Social Welfare had begun serious undertakings in this field as early as 1949. Using the slogan "We Have Added Years to Life—Now We Must Add Life to Years," the Department began to hold discussions with local authorities to encourage community services for the aged in the fields of employment, education, recreation, medical services, and the like.[35] In 1951 a state conference on aging, called by Governor Warren and attended by some 2,500 Californians, focused much of its attention on community efforts.[36] By 1959, the first year of the Brown administration, the Social Welfare Department had a firmly established community services program, and in 1961 this program was enormously expanded by the passage of Senate Bill 437.[37] In 1962 Congress passed a law providing matching funds for community service projects, and with this stimulus such projects have mushroomed in dozens of California communities.[38] If such efforts to educate the public to the plight of the older age groups have not yet produced any major breakthroughs, they must still be considered an important beginning.

Furthermore, the state government has not been content merely to publicize the problems of the older age groups and to urge communities to do something about them, but has instituted a number of tangible programs of its own. It has begun (but only begun) to deal with the problem of aged unemployment by legislating against employment discrimination on account of age, by providing employment and retraining services for the older worker, and by cooperating with private organizations to solve unemployment problems.[39] Some progress has been made in providing for the intellectual and psychological needs of retired persons by the expansion of adult education and library services.[40] And most important, the state has worked in fairly close conjunction with the federal government to devise solutions to problems of human aging that are obviously national in scope.

As already indicated, the Social Security system has generally brought a positive response in California, and many California officials would probably welcome having the entire state pension program placed under Society Security and funded by federal taxes.[41] Since 1964 the California League of Senior Citizens has been agitating for a national guaranteed annual pension for the aged, the blind, and the disabled, and this proposal has also gained rather wide endorsement from various leaders of public opinion in the state.[42] In 1965 Congress enacted a food stamp program for low-income families (a plan George McLain had proposed as early as 1951), and the California legislature voted to participate in it.[43] Although the effectiveness of the plan has been somewhat limited by the reluctance of various counties to participate, it has recently gained wide acceptance, often to the significant benefit of the older age groups.[44] Also in 1965 Congress passed the Older Americans Act, which created an Administration of Aging within the Department of Health, Education, and Welfare and provided grants-in-aid to states for various programs of aged aid.[45] California expanded its already extensive community services program under this act, and in 1969 the state's conservative United States Senator, George Murphy, apparently sensing its popularity, introduced legislation to extend the life of the act another three years.[46]

But the most important product of the coalition between California and the federal government on behalf of the aged has been the revolution in medical care and health services. The state began to deal with the problem on its own in the 1940's, when the legislature began to make appropriations for pensioners in county medical institutions and to expand the special-needs provision of the Old-Age Security Act to cover private medical care of many kinds.[47] But not until the middle 1950's was there a true appreciation of the problem. In 1955 an official report declared:

The medical needs of Old-Age Security recipients and the manner of meeting them constitute a problem which is increasingly predominant. . . . Aged persons, generally, have extensive health needs. There is growing recognition that they are entitled to receive and can use, with profit to the general welfare, a type of constructive medical care which goes beyond the merely palliative. There is much evidence, both nationally and within the State, of public interest in seeing that aged recipients of public assistance have the means to secure some measure at least, of the medical care that they need.[48]

The legislature's immediate response to this plea, though positive, was strictly traditional.[49] By 1957, however, some genuine innovations were introduced. In that year the legislature, responding to changes made by Congress in the Social Security Act in 1956, passed a law inaugurating the Public Assistance Medical Care program (PAMC). This law made state and federal funds available for outpatient services for the aged; in 1959 and 1960 it was amended to increase the maximum allocations for such services.[50] In 1961 California, again following the cue of Congress, which had just passed the Kerr-Mills Act, passed the Burton-Rattigan Act, which set up the program of Medical Assistance for the Aged (MAA). This program, which was 50 per cent funded by federal Kerr-Mills grants, provided hospital, nursing-home, and outpatient care to persons aged 65 or over who were defined as "medically indigent," i.e. capable of supporting themselves under ordinary circumstances but not under circumstances of prolonged illness.[51] Despite its many shortcomings, this program brought improved medical care to thousands of aged Californians.*

Probably of equal significance was the passage by Congress of the Community Health Services and Facilities Act in 1961, mak-

* The major shortcomings were a humiliating means test, a requirement that pensioners give up OAS benefits while receiving MAA funds, and the fact that MAA funds were available only after 30 days of hospitalization. The last shortcoming was corrected by the California legislature in 1963. Margaret Greenfield, *Medicare and Medicaid: The 1965 and 1967 Social Security Amendments* (Berkeley, Calif., 1968), pp. 13–14, 47, 64–71; *Maturity*, Sept. 1962.

ing federal funds available to state health departments for out-of-hospital health services to the chronically ill and aging. California enrolled in the program the following year, and the California State Department of Public Health immediately set up a Chronic Illness and Aging unit to coordinate local efforts and disburse funds.[52] The program has made available to the aged a broad range of health services, notably nursing-home care, home nursing, homemaking assistance, health aids, friendly visitors, telephone checks, and shopping services.[53]

But unquestionably the most important advance in medical services for the California aged has been the Medicare and Medi-Cal breakthrough of 1965. In that year Congress passed the Medicare and Medicaid acts, which provided extensive hospital and post-hospital care under the Social Security Act and enabled states to broaden their services to the "medically needy" of all ages who were not covered by Social Security.[54] There seems little question that Medicare has brought massive improvements in the economic and physical well-being of aged persons all over the United States.[55] It is quite possible, however, that the less-publicized Medicaid system will prove more far-reaching in its consequences, since it provides for the medically needy of all ages.[56]

In California the Medicaid system came into existence as the Medi-Cal Act of 1965. Although the law provides for a broad range of medical, hospital, post-hospital, and psychiatric care for beneficiaries of the state's programs of Aid to the Blind, Aid to the Disabled, Aid to Families with Dependent Children, and medical indigents of many kinds, most Medi-Cal beneficiaries are OAS recipients.[57] Recent surveys indicate that persons aged 65 or over are using Medi-Cal services at about twice the rate of those under 65 and that the annual average cost for the older age groups is nearly double the cost for the younger.[58] In fiscal 1968–69 the average monthly Medi-Cal payment for aged persons was $63.92, and the total Medi-Cal payment for them was $276,133,100—remarkably high expenditures when compared to the current average OAS cash grant of $103.62 and the total OAS cash grant disbursements of $374,682,100.[59]

The Medi-Cal Act, of course, has its defects; probably the most serious is that the "medically indigent" receive fewer benefits than those who are on some form of "categorical aid," such as an old-age pension.[60] On balance, however, it seems safe to say that the act's defects are vastly outweighed by its virtues. Studies indicate that Medi-Cal has greatly increased the availability of medical services, especially from the private sector of medical practice, and that it has widely expanded the number of eligible beneficiaries, centralized the administration of public medical care under state auspices, and brought property-tax relief to California localities.[61]

Medi-Cal had been vigorously pushed by both Governor Brown and George McLain, but McLain died shortly before its passage and Brown went out of office in the following year. The older age groups soon found reason to lament their passing from the political scene. Some of the dynamism of McLain's organization seems to have been lost with his death, although under his successors the California League of Senior Citizens has been reasonably active. The same can hardly be said for the old-age movement under Brown's successor, for Ronald Reagan has unquestionably proved a great disappointment to many of California's old people. Although a considerable percentage of them apparently voted for him in 1966, he soon became their primary political *bête noire*.[62] Beginning in 1967, CLSC spokesmen regularly referred to him as "Ron-the-Robber" and the "Jack-the-Ripper of Politics"; they castigated his political ambitions as "Reagomania" and asserted that his political philosophy can be summarized as "Go Beggin' with Reagan."[63] "He does not seem to care one little bit how much suffering he causes," Myrtle Williams has charged; "Governor Reagan has done more to harm our senior citizens than any other governor in California's history."[64]

Since the CLSC strongly supported Brown for reelection in 1966, some of this rhetoric can be attributed to political partisanship.[65] Still, it is a fact that Governor Reagan has demonstrated little enthusiasm for the political goals of the aged. Although the older age groups have made some advances during his administration, particularly in the areas of tax relief and broadened employment opportunities, on balance his record is negative, especially when compared with that of his predecessors.[66]

It is not that Reagan has anything against old people as such. It is simply that he is committed to a conservative political philosophy, which fears "big government," denigrates government "handouts" and social welfare programs, and gives top priority to lowering taxes and reducing spending. "Nothing is more important than reducing the cost of government," Reagan has frequently asserted, and his consistent adherence to this doctrine has had predictable effects on old-age politics in the state.*

From the old people's point of view, the Reagan administration's penchant for not only standing still but reverting to the welfare policies of decades past has proved a formidable obstacle to progress. Whereas they could once confine their efforts to prodding the legislature into liberalizing the Old-Age Security Act, under Reagan they have sometimes had to fight just to keep the status quo. Perhaps the bitterest conflict has been the dispute over the Social Security "pass-on." This controversy originated when the 1965 Congress raised OASI benefits by 7 per cent but failed to require states that supplemented OASI payments with state pensions to pass on this increase to pensioners. California, being one of those states that had many pensioners receiving OASI allowances supplemented by additional OAS grants, simply deducted the OASI increase from the OAS allowance, leaving the total cash grant the same as before and diverting the increased funds from the federal government into the state's general fund.[67] This policy seemed unfair and discriminatory to many, since it did not apply to those who were only on OASI. Accordingly Governor Brown, who had originally sanctioned the state's recapture of these funds, reversed himself and included the Social Security pass-on in his 1966–67 budget.[68]

Alas for the jubilant elders, this was a short-lived victory, for Governor Reagan struck the pass-on provision from his 1967–68 budget.[69] Although the legislature sided with the old people on this issue and passed a bill to carry out the pass-on principle and

* Los Angeles *Times*, Oct. 31, Sept. 18, 1969. For further indications of the Governor's feelings on this matter, particularly as it relates to public assistance expenditures, see *ibid.*, Oct. 29, 1969, and his budget messages in his proposed budgets for 1967–68, pp. v-xii, 1968–69, pp. v-xii, 1969–70, pp. vii-x; Calif. [11], pp. 12, 14–15; and San Gabriel Valley *Tribune*, Feb. 5, 1968. Governor Reagan seems to have moderated his views on fiscal matters recently, at least in his official rhetoric. His recent pronouncements indicate that he regards such matters as halting environmental pollution as more important than reduced spending, and his change of heart regarding state withholding taxes may also reflect a less rigidly conservative stance. Such a shift of position, if real rather than merely rhetorical, has had no discernible effect on his attitudes toward the older age groups, however.

to make it apply automatically to all future OASI increases, the Governor vetoed this measure. He also vetoed a second pro-aged bill that would have eliminated deductions for home-occupancy value from OAS checks.[70] In 1968, when the legislature again passed both bills, they were once again vetoed by the Governor; and his will prevailed, although the pass-on bill came closer than any other during his tenure thus far to being reenacted over his veto.[71] Since Congress had voted a new 13 per cent increase in Social Security benefits in 1967, this quarrel was more bitter than the first: there was, and is, more at stake for pensioners. The CLSC has continued to wage an incessant battle for the pass-on principle both in Sacramento and in Washington.*

Equally galling to the aged in California has been Reagan's economy drive against public health programs for low-income residents. Here, however, the older age groups and other opponents of the Governor seem to have been more successful in combating his policies. His notorious budget reductions in the Department of Mental Hygiene in 1967 had serious consequences for aged psychiatric patients, among others, and the furious opposition he faced from the CLSC and other quarters apparently persuaded the Governor to modify his stand in the following years.[72] Similarly, Reagan appeared convinced early in his administration that the Medi-Cal program would prove astronomically expensive and had to be curtailed.[73] Early in 1967 he instituted a policy of eliminating selected items from the program, such as eyeglasses, certain drugs, and surgical operations that doctors considered desirable but not absolutely necessary. The policy was described by the CLSC as "In other words: what's a little pain?" A storm of opposition arose from every quarter of the state, culminating in a state Supreme Court decision invalidating the Governor's cuts as contrary to law.[74] He nevertheless persisted in his efforts to have the Medi-Cal program curtailed, arguing that its costs were skyrocketing beyond the fiscal ability of the state to cover them, and being just as per-

---

* *Social Security Unemployment Compensation*, p. 32,058; *Senior Citizens Sentinel*, Feb., Mar., Apr., July, Oct., Nov. 1969. The 1969 Congress did pass a limited version of the pass-on principle. It raised Social Security benefits by 15 per cent and required that at least four dollars per month of this increase be passed on to OASI-OAS recipients. The CLSC understandably has hailed this as a great victory. *Senior Citizens Sentinel*, Feb. 1970.

sistently refuted by his own State Controller, who demonstrated in 1969 not only that the program was adequately funded but that both the Medi-Cal fund and the state treasury were showing substantial surpluses.[75]

In 1968 and 1969 the Governor continued to infuriate spokesmen for the aged by seeking the passage of laws to require most Medi-Cal recipients to pay 20 per cent of the program's cost,* to reinstitute property liens against public-assistance recipients, and to introduce a relative-responsibility clause into the Medi-Cal Act.[76] None of these measures was passed, however, and the CLSC took credit for "stop[ping] the Reagan poorhouse program dead in its tracks." In noting the Governor's expressed displeasure over the failures of certain proposals, spokesmen for the CLSC remarked, "The League is happy to have contributed to his disappointment."[77] The open warfare between the Governor and the CLSC continued to rage amid specific charges that the Governor was reducing OAS grants by administrative fiat[78] and general charges that he had revived the stereotype of the old-age pensioner as a sponger and a wastrel—a notion that was being combated and discredited as far back as the 1930's.[79] As of 1970, the bitterness of the anti-Reagan sentiment among California's economically deprived old people seemed boundless.

It would, nevertheless, be both inaccurate and unjust to lay all of the problems besetting California's old people at Reagan's door. As this study indicates, the problems of aging are endemic in modern society, and although California has wrestled energetically and often effectively with them over the past forty years, she has not eliminated those problems from her public life. The comparative poverty of old people relative to the rest of society obtains in California as well as in the rest of the nation, and it continues to be

* Senator John Harmer, who sponsored this proposal, sought to justify it as a measure to guard against the abuse of the law by people who allegedly use Medi-Cal services unnecessarily. "With some people, going to the doctor has become something of an indoor sport. It's the way they get their entertainment," the Senator reportedly once said. *Senior Citizens Sentinel*, Aug. 1969. This assertion is refuted by a state investigative report indicating that medical "shopping," along with the overuse of Medi-Cal services, is hardly a discernible problem. California, Office of Health Care Services, *Medical Care Resources and Utilization Project Report No. 5: Shopping for Medical Care by Welfare Recipients in Alameda County*.

intensified by employment discrimination.[80] Economic deprivation in turn continues to intensify physical and mental health
problems. Despite the great improvements wrought by Medicare
and Medi-Cal, many aged Californians suffer from chronic mala-
dies because they cannot afford adequate medical and psychiatric
treatment.[81] Furthermore, by its emphasis on post-hospital care
and the marginal adequacy of its allowances, Medi-Cal may actually be subsidizing a burgeoning growth of substandard nursing
homes that exploit and mistreat their aged charges instead of ministering effectively to their needs.[82]

In fact, not only nursing homes but homes in general are the
subject of one of the most basic controversies about aging in con-
temporary California and American life—a controversy that ex-
tends deep into the academic world. The traditional view, still
widely held, is that economic deprivation among the aged creates
a grave housing problem because it forces them to live in slums.[83]
Furthermore, this argument proceeds, even relatively affluent and
healthy old people tend to be forced out of the mainstream of society into special housing districts and retirement communities
where, deprived of their former social roles, they vegetate and de-
cay.[84] Even the elegant furnishings of Del Webb's Sun Cities and
Ross Cortesi's Leisure World colonies in Arizona and Southern
California are dysfunctional and repellent according to this view:
"The presence of death hangs almost daily over the retirement village like the effigy of an executed traitor."[85] Furthermore, the opu-
lence of the surroundings serves mainly to underline the hostility
and alienation of affluent old people forced into a purposeless existence. "The last cold defiance of the affluent aged is their possession of money they can't use. It is their measure—their only
remaining measure—of value in society. By denying it to society,
to charities, or to relatives they show their power."[86]

Although such rhetoric is compelling, there are good reasons to
doubt its accuracy. Over 80 per cent of America's old people, for
example, live not in tenements but in homes they or their spouses
own.[87] If their homes are not luxurious, they are hardly slums
in most cases. When interviewed by opinion samplers, only from
5 to 15 per cent of the aged complain about their housing arrange-
ments.[88] Moreover, there is a growing body of evidence that segre-
gation into boarding homes, retirement communities, or urban

neighborhoods provides old people with important services and affords them social and psychological satisfactions through being with other old people that are largely unattainable from society at large.[89] Perhaps it is pertinent that the California League of Senior Citizens, an organization closely in touch with the aspirations of its aged constituents and one hardly likely to deliberately exacerbate their plight, has established and maintains one successful Senior Citizens Village in Fresno and seeks to establish others.[90] If the housing problem of California's old people has not been solved, it is probably safe to say that this problem is far less pressing than others.

In fact it is probably still true that the most pressing problems of the California aged are more social than economic in character. Notwithstanding the disengagement hypothesis, the expulsion of the older age groups from active roles in American society seems to be accompanied by massive dissatisfactions and resentments. When a previously active person is required suddenly to face "the 'roleless role' of the retired in our society," he usually suffers considerable emotional distress.[91] Very likely the stress would be eased and the process of painless disengagement would be facilitated if mandatory retirement were accompanied with more respect, finesse, and economic aid from society at large. To be sure, in California the process has probably been eased somewhat because the state has led the way in economic support programs and Californians have been perhaps more sympathetic to the plight of the discontented aged than most Americans.[92] Nevertheless, social tensions remain acute enough to make one wonder whether the enlightened attitude of the California public is not a mere rhetorical posture. Perhaps the aspirations of the aged for acceptance and participation are merely given lip service by cynical politicians and a fundamentally heedless public.

On May 9, 1969, for example, Governor Reagan, while proclaiming the month of May as Senior Citizens Month, saw fit to refer to "senior Californians" as "one of the Golden State's most valuable resources, actively contributing to all segments of society." The aged, he added, "continue to provide us with a wealth of guidance and counsel born of the wisdom and experience of their years."[93] Straining awkwardly after further superlatives, the Governor went on to say:

The many working years of the senior Californian are the basis of the prosperity that all generations of Californians now enjoy, and they [sic] deserve the recognition of that merit; and ... every Californian will benefit from expanding the opportunities for the senior Californians to make fuller use of his [sic] talents and experience.

The fact that this classic articulation of the traditional rhetoric and ideology of the older age groups came from a public official who was at the very time "expanding the opportunities for the senior Californians" by withholding their Social Security increases and attempting to raise their medical bills dramatically demonstrates the gap between the real and the ideal in California old-age politics.

The Governor, it should be noted, is by no means the only Californian whose sensitivity to the problems of the aged is questionable. Other public officials have deplored what they regard as an overemphasis on aid to the aged at the expense of needy youth; private citizens have advocated giving the vote to eighteen-year-olds and denying it to persons over 65.[94] Furthermore, some state and county welfare officials continually advocate a return to property liens and strengthened relative-responsibility provisions for OAS recipients, oppose efforts to simplify OAS procedures by shifting the administration and financing of the program to the state level, insist on having the authority to give lie-detector tests to welfare applicants, and refuse to appoint welfare recipients to local poverty boards because they allegedly do not "have the intelligence to present a reasonable point of view."[95]

If California has dealt with the problems of aging, then, she has not solved them. She has not complied with the prescriptions of the activity theorists by giving old people active social roles; to achieve this goal, indeed, would require no less than a massive reordering of society. Nor has California been sufficiently adept in creating the general conditions wherein the older age groups can voluntarily disengage from society and continue to live meaningful and personally satisfying lives. No doubt some well-to-do old people have been able to achieve this gratifying position, but the vast majority of pensioners seem still to be living in a limbo of social and economic deprivation. So long as this situation continues, old-age politics can be expected to remain a prominent feature of the California scene.

Notes

Notes

Full authors' names, titles, and publication data for works cited in the Notes will be found in the Bibliography, pp. 191–204. Government publications are identified in the Notes and Bibliography by bracketed numbers and are listed in the Bibliography under California and United States. The following abbreviations are used in the Notes:

AAOAS: American Association for Old-Age Security

AB: Assembly Bills

Fin. Cal.: Final Calendar of Legislative Business

FOE: Fraternal Order of Eagles

JA: Journal of the Assembly

JS: Journal of the Senate

SB: Senate Bills

CHAPTER 1

1. World Almanac, 1969 (New York, 1969), pp. 606, 608, 593.

2. Population of California, p. 12; U.S. [4], p. xxxix.

3. Albrecht, "Sociological Impact of Aging," p. 1123; Birren and Bengston, p. 84; U.S. [19].

4. Statistics taken or computed from U.S. [1], Vol. II, pp. 154, 155, 194; U.S. [2], "Population," Vol. II, pp. 576–77, Vol. III, Pt. I, p. 234; U.S. [3], "Population," Vol. II, pp. 10, 519. The designation "aged" or "old" in this paragraph means persons aged 55 or over as well as those aged 65 or over.

5. Computed from U.S. [1], Vol. II, p. 362; U.S. [2], "Population," Vol. II, p. 591; U.S. [3], "Characteristics of the Population," Vol. II, pp. 23, 24, 123, 126, 136–37, 520, 523, 603–13, 629–57. See also Population of California, p. 208.

6. In 1960 persons who were 65 or over constituted 8.8 per cent of the total California population, whereas the percentage was 9.1 for the nation at large. Albrecht, "Sociological Impact of Aging," p. 1124; Goldstein, p. 454.

7. Population of California, pp. 55–58; Price, pp. 103–4.

8. Price, pp. 85–92.

9. McWilliams, Southern California Country, pp. 166–71.

10. *Ibid.*, pp. 171–75.

11. Havighurst and Albrecht, pp. 10–30.

12. Holtzman, "Analysis of Old-Age Politics," pp. 56–58; Harold E. Smith, "Family Interaction Patterns of the Aged: A Review," in Rose and Peterson, p. 153.

13. Havighurst, "Social and Psychological Needs"; Zinberg and Kaufman, pp. 33–40, 86–89.

14. Bond et al., pp. 296–300; Pinner et al., pp. 78–82; Shock, pp. 61–62; Touhy.

15. Pinner et al., p. 69; Talcott Parsons, "The Cultural Backgrounds of Today's Aged," in Donahue and Tibbitts, p. 3; Havighurst and Albrecht, p. 39; Walter G. Klopfer, "The Interpersonal Theory of Adjustment," in Kastenbaum, *Contributions,* pp. 37–43; Solomon; Kent; Ludwig and Eichorn.

16. Havighurst and Albrecht, p. 186; Bond et al., pp. 283–84, 287; Pinner et al., pp. 61–63, 68–69; Norman E. Zinberg and Irving Kaufman, "Culture and Personality Factors Associated with Aging: An Introduction," in Zinberg and Kaufman, p. 62. For contrary evidence on the effects of segregated housing on the aged see Rosow, pp. 35–40, 71–101, *passim.*

17. Epstein, *Insecurity,* p. 494; Martin and De Gruchy, p. 66; *Workers over 40;* U.S. [10], pp. 53–54; U.S. [16], pp. 19–23; Berwick.

18. Friedman and Havighurst, pp. 4, 7, 184; Kutner et al., pp. 78, 89–90; Zinberg and Kaufman, "Culture and Personality Factors," in Zinberg and Kaufman, pp. 45–56; Albrecht, "Sociological Impact of Aging"; Blau, pp. 29–31, 147–50, 152.

19. Epstein, "Old-Age Pensions," p. 226.

20. Epstein, *Insecurity,* p. 500; Lubove, pp. 134–35; Stewart, p. 4; Holtzman, "Townsend Movement" (diss.), p. 28; U.S. [13], p. 4.

21. U.S. [16], pp. 9–11; Goldstein, p. 455; U.S. [19], pp. vii–ix, xii–xiii, xviii–xix, 5, 7–8, 11–12, 27.

22. Epstein, *Challenge of the Aged,* pp. 93–112; Leven et al., pp. 54, 87; Beman, pp. 30, 60–61; Lubove, pp. 124–32; Nelson, pp. 56–57; U.S. [13], p. 19; Clague, p. 346; Epstein, "Sidelight on the Family Status," p. 31.

23. Holtzman, "Townsend Movement" (diss.), p. 17; Martin A. Berezin, "Some Intrapsychic Aspects of Aging," in Zinberg and Kaufman, pp. 107–10.

24. *Support of the Aged,* p. 12; Arthur M. Schlesinger, Jr., *The Coming of the New Deal* (Boston, 1959), p. 31.

25. U.S. [9], p. 4; Harry C. Evans, "The American Poorhouse," in Beman, p. 106; Epstein, *Facing Old Age,* pp. 30, 59; Epstein, *Insecurity,* p. 501; Lubove, pp. 132–34.

26. Epstein, "Present Status of Old-Age Pension Legislation," pp. 761–62; Epstein, *Facing Old Age,* pp. 13–16; Kutner et al., p. 90; U.S. [13], p. 43; U.S. [16], p. 12. One authority even asserts that physicians have certain psychological inhibitions toward aged patients and give them less

than adequate therapy for this reason. See Alvin I. Goldfarb, "A Psychosocial and Sociophysiological Approach to Aging," in Zinberg and Kaufman, pp. 85–86.

27. On the relationship between social deprivation and failing mental health in the aged, see Martin and De Gruchy, p. 65; Kutner et al., pp. 78–81, 89–90; Albrecht, "Social Roles of Old People"; George A. Sacher, "On Longevity Regarded as Organized Behavior: The Role of Brain Structure," in Kastenbaum, *Contributions*, pp. 99–110; Alvin I. Goldfarb, "A Psychosocial and and Sociophysiological Approach to Aging," in Zinberg and Kaufman, p. 80; and Martin A. Berezin, "Some Intrapsychic Aspects of Aging," in Zinberg and Kaufman, pp. 94–95. On relationships between failing physical and failing mental health, see Zinberg and Kaufman, pp. 23–32, and Preston, p. 201.

28. On the therapeutic value of social participation to the aged see Gilbert, pp. 322–25, 328–32; Martin A. Berezin, "Some Intra-psychic Aspects of Aging," in Zinberg and Kaufman, pp. 113–17; and Stokes and Maddox. On the particular fitness of aged persons for advisory roles see Martin and De Gruchy, pp. 9–23; Schramm and White; Berelson et al., pp. 25, 91–92; Crittenden, "Aging and Political Participation"; Rosow, pp. 10–13; and Glenn. For some contrary evidence see Pollak; Gergen and Back; Rosenblatt; and Thune et al.

29. Drake, p. 79; Gilbert, pp. 56–66; "Gerontion"; Havighurst, "Social and Psychological Needs," pp. 15–16; Maurice E. Linden, "Regression and Recession in the Psychoses of the Aging," in Zinberg and Kaufman, pp. 125–42.

30. Pinner et al., p. 69.

31. For detailed statistical evidence see Putnam, "Influence of the Older Age Groups," pp. 29–32; and see also Calif. [14] and [15].

32. For some sociological and psychological evidence of the tendency of groups and individuals to anticipate sharing the fate of others see Robert Merton, *Social Theory and Social Structure* (Glencoe, Ill., 1957), pp. 265–68; and Norman E. Zinberg and Irving Kaufman, "Culture and Personality Factors," in Zinberg and Kaufman, pp. 45–46.

33. Heller Committee, pp. 2, 48; Calif. [24], 1927–28, p. 163; Dodd and Penrose, pp. 93–96; Bond et al., pp. 280–81; Pinner et al., p. 59.

34. Pinner et al., pp. 62, 67–68; Bond et al., p. 288; Martin and De Gruchy, p. 13; Schramm and Storey, pp. 72–91.

35. For arguments supporting the uniqueness of old-age politics in the United States see Lloyd H. Fisher, "The Politics of Age," in Derber, pp. 165–66; Holtzman, "Analysis of Old-Age Politics," pp. 56–58; and Philibert, pp. 5–6.

36. Barron.

37. Lloyd H. Fisher, "The Politics of Age," in Derber, pp. 163–65; Pinner et al., pp. 2, 91.

38. Cresap, pp. 36–37; Jacobs and Gallagher, pp. 104–6; Crouch et al., chap. 4; McWilliams, *California*, pp. 207–13.

39. James Q. Wilson, "The Political Culture of Southern California,"

Commentary, May 1967, reprinted in Dennis Hale and Jonathan Eisen, eds., *The California Dream* (New York, 1968), p. 228. See also Bond et al., pp. 265–66, 269.

40. Pinner et al., pp. 56–60, 62–63; Bond et al., p. 285; Lloyd H. Fisher, "The Politics of Age," in Derber, p. 163; Holtzman, "Townsend Movement" (diss.), p. 264; Neuberger and Loe, pp. 12–13.

41. Pinner et al., pp. 1–13; Lane, p. 168; Cantril, pp. 185–89, 201–9; Mannheim; Rudolf Heberle, *Social Movements: An Introduction to Political Sociology* (New York, 1951), chap. 6.

42. Barron, pp. 477–78; Pinner et al., pp. 6–7; Cantril, pp. 201–9; Lane, p. 159; Schmidhauser, "Political Influence of the Aged."

43. Pinner et al., p. 91; Barron; Lipset, p. 269; Campbell et al., p. 357.

44. See statements by pension spokesman in "What Price Old Age Security?" p. 372.

45. Glane, pp. 124–28; Pinner et al., pp. 23–27, 71.

46. *Modern Crusader,* Sept. 29, 1934, p. 6.

47. Carlson, p. 173.

48. Pinner et al., pp. 78–82. Despite its troublesome side effects, this provision still has widespread public support. A survey taken in 1960 showed that although nine out of ten adults thought aged parents should not live with their children, a majority thought that the children rather than the government should care for aged parents who were in economic need. Morgan, pp. 3–4.

49. Brief delineations of this theory and some of its implications can be found in Kleemeier; Harry Sobel, "Aging Theory: Cellular and Extracellular Modalities," in Kastenbaum, *Contributions,* pp. 57–67; and Alvin I. Goldfarb, "A Psychosocial and Sociophysiological Approach to Aging," in Zinberg and Kaufman, p. 77.

50. For a sophisticated use of this kind of approach see Blau, pp. 87–90. See also M. Elaine Cumming, "New Thoughts on the Theory of Disengagement," in Kastenbaum, *New Thoughts,* pp. 4–7.

51. Lane, pp. 151–68, 218–19.

52. At the present time women constitute about 57 per cent of the 65-and-over population in the United States, and this percentage will undoubtedly increase. U.S. [19], p. 3.

53. This analysis is taken from Kent, pp. 682–83, and from Norman E. Zinberg and Irving Kaufman, "Culture and Personality Factors," in Zinberg and Kaufman, p. 49.

54. This theory was first presented in Cumming and Henry. For elaborations and refinements see Havighurst, "Social-Psychological Perspective"; M. Elaine Cumming, "New Thoughts on the Theory of Disengagement," in Kastenbaum, *New Thoughts,* pp. 3–18; William E. Henry, "Engagement and Disengagement: Toward a Theory of Adult Development," in Kastenbaum, *Contributions,* pp. 19–35; Robert Kastenbaum, "Engrossment and Perspective in Later Life: A Developmental Field Approach," in Kastenbaum, *Contributions,* pp. 3–18; Kastenbaum, "Theories of Human Aging," pp. 23–36; and Kleemeier.

55. Some interesting attempts in this regard are Havighurst, "Social-Psychological Perspective," p. 68; William E. Henry, "Engagement and Disengagement: Toward a Theory of Adult Development," in Kastenbaum, *Contributions,* pp. 19–35; M. Elaine Cumming, "New Thoughts on the Theory of Disengagement," in Kastenbaum, *New Thoughts,* pp. 4–6; and Mercer and Butler.

56. Cumming and Henry, p. 33.

57. Arnold M. Rose, "The Subculture of Aging: A Framework for Research in Social Gerontology," in Rose and Peterson, pp. 3–16. For further evidence of the relative success of the older age groups in establishing meaningful community life in separate communities see Rosow, *passim.* This increase in affluence should not be overemphasized, since the overall financial condition of the older age groups is still poor by most national standards. In fact, their situation tends to worsen in comparison with that of the rest of the population and may well continue to do so in the future. U.S. [19], pp. 27–39. Compared to their plight in earlier decades, however, the economic condition of the older age groups seems to have improved remarkably.

CHAPTER 2

1. Calif. [24], July 1938–June 1940, pp. 19–20; Bond et al., pp. 41–44.

2. Bond et al., pp. 44–45; Cahn and Bary, pp. 146, 172; Glane, p. 51.

3. As late as 1932 a welfare official in Merced County demanded that the state "grant old-age aid to those whose lives prove that they have made an effort in life.... Otherwise send them to the poorhouse even though it should cost more." U.S. [18], pp. 11–12.

4. There were 62 county poorhouses in the state in 1920 and 73 in 1930. The number of inmates increased from 6,961 to 15,372. Calif. [1], July 1918–June 1920, p. 13; Calif. [24], July 1928–June 1930, p. 46. There was an even larger increase in the number of state-licensed nursing or boarding homes for the aged, many of which were supported by private charities. Calif. [19], pp. 153–55; Calif. [24], 1927–28, p. 98, and July 1930–June 1932, pp. 65, 71.

5. Harry C. Evans, "The American Poorhouse," in Beman, p. 106; U.S. [9]; Lubove, pp. 132–34; Cahn and Bary, pp. 148–51.

6. Epstein, *Insecurity,* p. 501, and *Facing Old Age,* p. 30; Calif. [24], 1927–28, pp. 137, 187; Heller Committee, pp. 1, 23.

7. Calif. [1], July 1918–June 1920, p. 132; Calif. [24], 1927–28, pp. 164, 187, and July 1938–June 1940, p. 20.

8. Calif. [24], 1927–28, p. 187.

9. This blunder is probably as much the fault of professional social workers as of callous politicians. In 1901 the first statewide organization of social workers was founded under the name California State Conference of Charities and Corrections. It changed its name to California State Conference of Social Agencies in 1911, however, and is known today as the California Association of Health and Welfare. Bornet, *Welfare in America,* pp. 236–37.

10. Calif. [19], p. 9; Bond et al., p. 68.

11. For evidence of the continuation of the Progressive movement in California into the 1920's and the merging of the business with the Progressive ethos see Putnam, "Persistence of Progressivism."

12. Bond et al., pp. 47–48; Calif. [1], July 1918–June 1920, and July 1920–June 1922, p. 120; Calif. [19], pp. 31–35.

13. Sacramento *Bee,* Jan. 18, Mar. 10, 1921, Feb. 1, Mar. 5, Mar. 10, Apr. 13, Apr. 14, 1923, Jan. 7, Jan. 13, 1925; Bond et al., pp. 51–52; Calif. [19], pp. 10–12.

14. Sacramento *Bee,* Apr. 4, 1927; Bond et al., p. 52; Calif. [24], 1927–28, p. 4.

15. Lubove, pp. 135–36; Le Brun, pp. 453–54.

16. Hansen, *The Eagles,* pp. 1–2.

17. Hansen, *Eagles Are People Helping People,* p. 8; FOE, *Historic Words,* preface; "California Triumphant," p. 6; Lubove, p. 137.

18. FOE, *Social Security,* p. 4.

19. Hansen, *Eagles Are People Helping People,* p. 8; Holtzman, "Analysis of Old-Age Politics," p. 59; Epstein, "Present Status of Old-Age Pension Legislation," p. 763; Lubove, p. 138.

20. Lubove, pp. 137–38; Hansen, *Eagles Are People Helping People;* FOE, *Answers to Objections;* Beman, pp. 151–65.

21. Lubove, pp. 114–19.

22. *Ibid.,* p. 139; Epstein, "Present Status of Old-Age Pension Legislation," pp. 765–66; Beman, pp. 300, 305.

23. Lubove, p. 138; Epstein, "Present Status of Old-Age Pension Legislation," pp. 763–64; "Old-Age Pension Bill."

24. Lubove, p. 136; Le Brun, pp. 453–58; FOE, *Social Security,* pp. 4–6; Epstein, "Present Status of Old-Age Pension Legislation," pp. 763–64; U.S. [11], pp. 1–2, 5–6.

25. Bond et al., p. 53.

26. "California Triumphant," p. 6.

27. *Ibid.;* Sacramento *Bee,* Jan. 18, 1923; Calif. [43], *JS,* 45th sess., 1923, p. 171; Sacramento *Bee,* Mar. 21, 1923; Calif. [42], *JA,* 45th sess., 1923, p. 205.

28. Calif. [42], *JA,* 45th sess., 1923, pp. 2050, 2199, 2596; Calif. [43], *JS,* 45th sess., 1923, pp. 1687–88, 1742, 1917–18; Calif. [41], *Fin. Cal.,* 45th sess., 1923, p. 139.

29. Herbert W. Slater, "Political Gossip," Santa Rosa *Press-Democrat,* Jan. 2, 1925.

30. Sacramento *Bee,* Mar. 7, 1925.

31. Frankhouser, pp. 372–74.

32. Walker and Cave, p. 191.

33. Sacramento *Bee,* Jan. 12, Jan. 14, Mar. 7, 1925; "California Triumphant," p. 6; Calif. [42], *JA,* 46th sess., 1925, p. 1856; Calif. [43], *JS,* 46th sess., 1925, p. 1753. The 1925 legislature was decidedly more progressive than that of 1923, which probably accounts for the easy passage of a pension bill almost identical to the one that had been watered down in the

earlier sessions and vetoed by the Governor. Putnam, "Persistence of Progressivism," pp. 406–7.

34. Calif. [42], *JA*, 46th sess., 1925, p. 2554.

35. Le Brun, p. 455; Roseman, p. 54; Lubove, p. 141; Calif. [40], *AB*, 1923, AB 309; Calif. [46], *SB*, 1923, SB 168; *Calif.* [40], *AB*, 1925, AB 4.

36. Holtzman, "Analysis of Old-Age Politics," p. 59; FOE, *Social Security*; Epstein, *Old-Age Security*, p. 34.

37. Putnam, "Persistence of Progressivism," pp. 408–11.

38. Long Beach *Press-Telegram*, Nov. 3, 1930; Pasadena *Star-News*, Oct. 31, 1930; Santa Cruz *News*, Nov. 21, 1929; letter from Governor Young to Will J. French, Director, Calif. Dept. of Industrial Relations, in Calif. [14], p. 7.

39. Evidence of the public's increasing awareness of the problems of old age is to be found in the Santa Rosa *Press-Democrat*, Apr. 2, 1921, and Aug. 3, 1922. For the establishment of the AAOAS chapter, see San Francisco *Chronicle*, Jan. 23, 1928.

40. Calif. [42], *JA*, 47th sess., 1927, pp. 336, 1832, 2551, 2653; Calif. [41], *Fin. Cal.*, 47th sess., 1927, p. 295.

41. Heller Committee, p. vii; Santa Rosa *Press-Democrat*, Feb. 2, 1928.

42. The tendency to investigate problems instead of acting on them is described, though not quite in these terms, by former State Senator Herbert C. Jones in his reminiscences, "On California Government and Public Issues," p. 97. The De Turbeville Report was quite widely circulated and was published in three different forms: Calif., *Appendix to the Journals of the Senate and Assembly*, 48th sess., 1929; Calif. [30]; and Calif. [24], 1927–28, pp. 158–219.

43. Calif. [24], 1927–28, pp. 164, 176–79, 180, 187, 199–200.

44. *Ibid.*, p. 166.

45. *Ibid.*, pp. 170–73.

46. *Ibid.*, pp. 182–83.

47. Calif. [42], *JA*, 48th sess., 1929, pp. 172, 145; Calif. [40], *AB*, 1929, AB 166, AB 1046; Sacramento *Bee*, Jan. 11, Feb. 20, 1929; "California Triumphant," p. 6.

48. "California Triumphant," p. 7; Sacramento *Bee*, Mar. 6, Mar. 21, 1929; Calif. [42], *JA*, 48th sess., 1929, p. 678.

49. Calif. [42], *JA*, 48th sess., 1929, pp. 1531, 2547; Calif. [43], *JS*, 48th sess., 1929, p. 2531; Calif. [41], *Fin. Cal.*, 48th sess., 1929, p. 132; "California Triumphant," pp. 5, 39; FOE, *Historic Words*, pp. 10–11; De Turbeville, pp. 292–93.

50. Actually, Wyoming had passed a mandatory law earlier in the year, but it did not go into effect until June 1, 1930, whereas California's became effective August 14, 1929, in the matter of receiving applications, with payments to begin January 1, 1930. *California Statutes*, 1929, chap. 530; "California Triumphant," pp. 5–6, 40.

51. *California Statutes*, 1929, chap. 530.

52. On September 23, 1929, Governor Young appointed Esther De Turbeville chief of the division. Miss De Turbeville died in the summer

of 1930. Olive Henderson, "One Year's Experience with Pensions in California," in AAOAS, *Fourth National Conference*, pp. 50–51; San Francisco *Chronicle*, Sept. 24, 1929, p. 12.

53. Bond et al., pp. xxi, 60; Andrews, p. 294; "California Old-Age Pension Law"; Rogers, p. 15; Le Brun, p. 456; Glane, p. 63; *Lake County Bee*, June 5, 1929; Long Beach *Press-Telegram*, Aug. 18, 1929, section C; Pasadena *Star-News*, Aug. 14, 1929; Redlands *Daily Facts*, Aug. 19, 1929; Santa Rosa *Press-Democrat*, May 29, June 14, 1929.

54. De Turbeville, p. 293. The same point was made by Governor Young when he signed the bill into law. FOE, *Historic Words*, pp. 10–11.

55. Carlson, p. 173.

56. Calif. [24], July 1934–June 1936 with additional data for July 1932–June 1934, between pp. 20–21; Peirce, p. 87.

57. Olive Henderson, "One Year's Experience with Pensions in California," in AAOAS, *Fourth National Conference*, p. 51; Bond et al., p. 59.

58. Holtzman, "Analysis of Old-Age Politics," p. 60; Peirce, p. 87.

59. Abraham Epstein asserted, perhaps somewhat overenthusiastically, that the 1929 law "makes it possible to maintain two persons on a pension for less than the cost of supporting one inmate in an almshouse." *Insecurity*, p. 544. He estimated the number of old people saved from the poorhouse by 1932 to be more than 4,000. "What Price Old-Age Security?" p. 342.

60. Epstein, *Insecurity*, p. 539. For further evidence of the emotional relief felt by pension recipients in California, see U.S. [18], pp. 7–8; Epstein, *Insecurity*, pp. 537–38; AAOAS, *Fourth National Conference*, pp. 52–53.

61. Holtzman, "Analysis of Old-Age Politics," p. 60.

62. Peirce, pp. 86, 88; U.S. [11], pp. 26, 28; Parker; U.S. [18], pp. 19, 35; Calif. [24], July 1930–June 1932, between pp. 22–23; Putnam, "Influence of the Older Age Groups," pp. 154–55.

63. U.S. [18], pp. 11–12.

64. "California Triumphant," p. 39; San Francisco *Chronicle*, June 14, 1937.

65. The statement on Hornblower's voice is from Patterson, p. 246. On Hornblower's connections with leading lobbyists, see Philbrick, Pt. II, pp. 3–23, 50–54, and Pt. IV, pp. 2–5; and Clark, pp. 87–88. Also associated with Hornblower both in his lobby connections and in his work on behalf of the aged was his fellow Eagle Assemblyman Charles W. Lyon. See Clark, pp. 87–88, and various ephemeras in the Charles W. Lyon Papers.

66. Calif. [40], *AB*, 1931, AB 76; Calif. [42] *JA*, 49th sess., 1931, pp. 319, 851, 1882, 1927, 2081, 2591, 3650, 3901; Calif. [43], *JS*, 49th sess., 1931, pp. 2014–15, 2244, 2279; Calif. [41], *Fin. Cal.*, 49th sess., 1931, p. 128; *California Statutes*, 1931, chap. 608.

67. AAOAS, *Fifth National Conference*, pp. 48–49.

68. U.S. [18], pp. 38–39.

69. Peirce, pp. 87, 88; Calif. [5], p. 1988.

70. Glane, pp. 112–13; Parker, p. 267.

71. Santa Rosa *Press-Democrat*, Oct. 17, 1931, p. 10; "What Price Old-Age Security?" pp. 339, 346–47, 353, 372.

72. "What Price Old-Age Security?" p. 372.

73. *Ibid.*, pp. 363–66.

74. *Ibid.*, pp. 371–72.

75. *Ibid.*, p. 351.

76. Olive Henderson, "Three Years of Old-Age Security in California," in AAOAS, *Sixth National Conference*, pp. 46–47; Henderson, "Four Years of Old-Age Security in California," in AAOAS, *Seventh National Conference*, p. 50.

77. Santa Rosa *Press-Democrat*, Dec. 16, 1932, Jan. 6, 1933; Sacramento *Bee*, Jan. 4, 1933.

78. Sacramento *Bee*, Jan. 5, 6, and 15, 1933. For other reactions against the proposal see *ibid.*, Jan. 20, Mar. 11, Mar. 18, 1933; Pasadena *Star-News*, Mar. 3, 1933. Rolph had campaigned on the slogan "Smile with Sunny Jim" in his successful bid for the governorship in 1930.

79. San Francisco *Chronicle*, Jan. 27, Feb. 1, 1933.

80. Sacramento *Bee*, Apr. 11, 1933; *Sacramento Union*, July 22, 26, and 27, 1933; Santa Rosa *Press-Democrat*, July 19, 1933; Calif. [24], July 1934–June 1936, p. 21.

81. Peirce, pp. 86, 89; Calif. [24], July 1934–June 1936, p. 21.

82. *Upton Sinclair's EPIC News*, June 4, 1934. That these reductions worked severe deprivations on many pensioners is evidenced by the fact that, according to at least one state hospital supervisor, pensioners often came there "showing effects of malnutrition and neglect." "What Price Old-Age Security?" p. 353.

83. Calif. [40], *AB*, 1933, AB 1778; *California Statutes*, 1933, chap. 761.

84. Calif. [42], *JA*, 50th sess., 1933, pp. 588, 589, 665, 4602, 4604, 4622–23; Glane, pp. 67–68.

85. Glane, pp. 67–68; Calif. [46], *SB*, 1933, SB 706; Calif. [43], *JS*, 50th sess., 1933, pp. 450, 3485.

86. Sacramento *Bee*, Mar. 23, 1933; Putnam, "Influence of the Older Age Groups," pp. 169–70.

CHAPTER 3

1. Caughey, pp. 49–50.

2. Cain, p. 280.

3. *Ibid.*, pp. 272–73.

4. Cleland, p. 212.

5. Cain, p. 272.

6. Cleland, pp. 212–13; McWilliams, *Southern California Country*, chap. 13.

7. Creel, *Rebel at Large*, p. 280.

8. Cleland, pp. 216–18; Whiteman and Lewis, chap. 11; McIntosh, pp. 99–104.

9. McIntosh, pp. 104–11; Cleland, pp. 219–20; Whiteman and Lewis, chaps. 3–4.

10. Creel, *Rebel at Large*, pp. 282–85; Whiteman and Lewis, chap. 3.

11. Whiteman and Lewis, chap. 18; McWilliams, *Southern California Country*, p. 302; McIntosh, pp. 75–83, 97–99.

12. Townsend, *Autobiography*, p. 170.

13. McIntosh, p. 4; Chinn, pp. 22–24; Larsen, pp. 127–32.

14. For some of the economically unsound features of Sinclair's program see Larsen, pp. 131–32. A different assessment is to be found in McIntosh, p. 13.

15. Burke, pp. 2–3; Creel, *Rebel at Large*, pp. 268–71; Chinn, pp. 14–15, 36–37; McIntosh, pp. 119–38.

16. Sinclair, *I, Candidate*, pp. 44–46; "The Lie Factory Starts," in Sinclair, *EPIC Plan*, pp. 18–27.

17. Cresap, p. 92. The most famous of Sinclair's tracts was entitled *I, Governor of California and How I Ended Poverty: A True Story of the Future*. Several other pamphlets are reprinted in Sinclair's *EPIC Plan for California*. More important, perhaps, was the party newspaper, called at various times *Upton Sinclair's End Poverty Paper, Upton Sinclair's EPIC News, National EPIC News*, and finally simply the *EPIC News*. Henceforth this newspaper will be referred to as the *EPIC News*.

18. Burke, p. 8; Sinclair, *I, Candidate*, p. 101; Chinn, pp. 39–43.

19. Cresap, p. 39; Whiteman and Lewis, p. 217; Alsop and Kintner, pp. 7, 85–86.

20. In an early editorial entitled "End Povery Is the Only Issue" Sinclair urged all EPIC speakers to "stick to the text" by merely asserting that they proposed to end poverty for all dissatisfied groups, even including the Nazi-admiring "Silver Shirts" and the antiprohibitionist "Wets," and not to be drawn into championing certain groups and antagonizing others. *EPIC News*, May 1934.

21. Sinclair, *I, Governor*, p. 38.

22. For examples of pension sentiment in the state at this time see San Andreas *Calaveras Prospect*, June 30, 1934; El Centro *Imperial Valley Press*, July 2, 1934; Napa *Journal*, Aug. 26, 1934; Pasadena *Star-News*, Aug. 7, 1934; Santa Rosa *Press-Democrat*, Aug. 9, 1934.

23. Chinn, p. 56. See also Larsen, p. 140; and McIntosh, pp. 183–94, 204–5.

24. Chinn, pp. 54–56.

25. See "The Lie Factory Starts," in Sinclair, *EPIC Plan*; Sinclair, *I, Governor*, pp. 118–72; Cleland, pp. 224–27; Caughey, pp. 517–18; Larsen, pp. 133–38, 147; McIntosh, pp. 227–66.

26. Max Stern in the San Francisco *News*, Nov. 2, 1934, quoted in Chinn, p. 104.

27. Sinclair, *I, Candidate*, chap. 36; Larsen, pp. 139–40.

28. Holtzman, "Townsend Movement" (diss.), pp. 36–37; Whiteman and Lewis, p. 224.

29. Pasadena *Star-News*, Oct. 27, 1934; Chinn, p. 57; California Democratic Party Platform, 1934, California State Library Collection of Campaign Literature. The state platform plank was a watered-down version of Sinclair's original old-age pension proposal. It called for only "ade-

quate" old-age pensions and said nothing about pensions of $50 a month. Ironically, both Creel and McAdoo were influential in securing a weakened version of the pension plank in the Democratic platform. McIntosh, pp. 179, 183, 189, 194, 196.

30. Sinclair, "Immediate EPIC," p. 26; *EPIC News*, Sept. 24, Oct. 1, 1934; Sinclair, *I, Candidate*, p. 97.

31. For a particularly adroit attack on Sinclair on this issue, see the Bakersfield *Californian*, Sept. 15, 1934.

32. Whiteman and Lewis, p. 219.

33. Long Beach *Press-Telegram*, Sept. 12, 1934; Chinn, p. 103; "Assembly Joint Resolution No. 1—Relative to Memorializing the President and Congress to Provide for Old Age Pensions," *Statutes of California*, 1935, chap. 1.

34. *EPIC News*, July 16, Aug. 25, 1934.

35. Chinn, p. 103; Whiteman and Lewis, p. 230; Alsop and Kintner, pp. 85–86.

36. *The EBIC Snooze*, Oct. 1, 1934. This publication was a Haight campaign newspaper, its title being an obvious satire on Sinclair's *EPIC News*. EBIC stood for "Expose Bunk in California." California State Library Collection of Campaign Literature. See also Sinclair, *I, Candidate*, p. 148.

37. Republican Party Platform, 1934, and Merriam Campaign leaflet, Bancroft Library Collection of Campaign Literature from the California Election of 1934.

38. Sinclair, *I, Candidate*, p. 97. Sinclair also pointed out, to no avail, that even the Republicans were not unanimous in their support of the Townsend plan, and that George Hatfield, the Republican nominee for lieutenant governor, was vociferously opposed to it. *EPIC News*, Oct. 8, 1934.

39. Holtzman, "Townsend Movement" (diss.), pp. 500–501; *Modern Crusader*, Sept. 29, Oct. 17, 1934. *The Modern Crusader* was the earliest Townsend organ. The October 16 issue carried a full-page political advertisement describing Sinclair as a radical and a free lover and declaring, "He pledged the people (in his Primary campaign) an old-age pension. Afterward he repudiated his promise." It closed with the flat assertion:

Sinclair IS NOT for the Townsend Plan
Merriam IS FOR the Townsend Plan.

40. McIntosh, p. 320. Sinclair might have been more successful had he continued to advocate state old-age pensions and either refused to commit himself on the merits of the Townsend plan or given a qualified endorsement of it, provided that a more equitable method of financing it were proposed. In later years Sinclair defended his outspoken and impolitic opposition to the plan on the ground that he was not really trying to get elected but only attempting to "educate the people" (*I, Candidate*, p. 98). This explanation seems dubious.

41. Chinn, p. 105; Calif. [53], General Election, Nov. 6, 1934, p. 5.

42. Calif. [53], General Election, Nov. 6, 1934, p. 6; Fitzgerald, p. 19. Downey's heavier vote can also be explained by the fact that there was no important third party in the contest for lieutenant governor as there was with Raymond Haight in the contest for governor.

43. These 23 persons were true EPIC men in that they ran under the EPIC label in the primary election. After the primary the EPIC organization endorsed all Democratic candidates for the Assembly in hopes that they would feel obligated to cooperate with the EPIC men if elected. Of this latter group 16 were elected, but they apparently did not feel obligated to cooperate with the EPIC organization at all. In fact, they "usually voted with the Republican majority in the Legislature against the original EPICs." Chinn, pp. 127–28.

44. Whiteman and Lewis, pp. 238–41; Sacramento *Union*, Jan. 15, Apr. 2, Apr. 8, Apr. 20, Apr. 25, June 4, 1935; Ford, pp. 11–12; McIntosh, p. 360.

45. *EPIC News*, July 22, 1935.

46. *Ibid.*, May 13, June 10, 1935; Sacramento *Union*, May 27, May 28, June 5, 1935.

47. Sacramento *Union*, June 5, June 14, 1935; *EPIC News*, Sept. 16, 1935.

48. *EPIC News*, Aug. 3, 1936.

49. *Ibid.*, Feb. 22, 1937.

50. *Ibid.*, Dec. 14, 1936.

51. *Ibid.*, Jan. 4, Feb. 15, 1937.

52. *Ibid.*, Mar. 29, Apr. 12, Apr. 19, Apr. 26, May 3, May 10, 1937.

53. *Ibid.*, Mar. 29, Apr. 26, May 31, June 21, Aug. 23, Nov. 1, 1937.

54. *Ibid.*, Dec. 13, Dec. 27, 1937, Jan. 3, 1938, Feb. 1, 1939, Sept. 1940, Jan. 1941. The EPIC organization exerted considerable pressure as well at the national level, especially through Los Angeles Congressman Jerry Voorhis, for more liberal pensions under the National Social Security Act. *Ibid.*, Feb. 4, Feb. 11, Oct. 28, 1935, June 21, Sept. 20, Nov. 8, Nov. 27, 1937, Aug. 29, 1938. Voorhis had been an unsuccessful EPIC candidate for the state legislature in 1934. Voorhis, pp. 17–19.

55. *EPIC News*, Sept. 16, 1935.

56. *Ibid.*, Feb. 4, 1935, Aug. 3, Aug. 17, 1936, Feb. 8, Mar. 22, Sept. 13, 1937, Feb. 15, 1940.

57. *Ibid.*, Jan. 21, 1935, Sept. 28, 1936, Feb. 15, Apr. 26, Sept. 29, Oct. 4, Oct. 11, Oct. 18, Nov. 29, Dec. 20, 1937, Jan. 10, Feb. 7, Feb. 21, Mar. 14, 1938.

58. *Ibid.*, Feb. 25, July 22, Oct. 14, 1935, June 22, Nov. 23, Dec. 14, 1936, Feb. 1, Mar. 29, June 21, June 28, 1937, Apr. 1, 1939.

59. *Ibid.*, Feb. 18, Mar. 11, Apr. 1, Apr. 15, 1935; Sacramento *Union*, Mar. 26, 1935; Fitzgerald, p. 20.

60. *EPIC News*, Apr. 8, 1935.

61. *Ibid.*

62. *National Townsend Weekly*, Apr. 15, 1935; Townsend, *Autobiography*, p. 170.

63. *EPIC News*, Nov. 11, 1935. See also *ibid.*, Mar. 23 and Apr. 6, 1936, for a fanciful and totally unworkable proposal of how to provide this $200 in goods and services or in cash (as the Townsend plan envisioned) to California's aged.

64. *Ibid.*, Oct. 28, Nov. 4, Apr. 27, 1935.

65. *Ibid.*, Dec. 2, 1935. The EPIC men had made other criticisms of the Townsend plan at the same time that they were courting the Townsendites. See especially an article by L. Raymond Holmes in *ibid.*, Oct. 21, 1935. Quite probably there was always a split in the ranks of the EPIC organization over the correct position to take in regard to the Townsend plan.

66. Whiteman and Lewis, p. 230.

67. Downey, *Why I Believe in the Townsend Plan*, pp. 92, 101–3, 105–6, 112–13.

68. *Ibid.*, p. 10.

69. *EPIC News*, Apr. 13, 1936. There were rumors that the Democrats planned to reward Downey for his "statesmanship" in trying to bring these two groups together by instituting a recall of Governor Merriam and running Downey as his successor. Downey coyly declared that he would "just as soon they'd leave me out of this" because he was devoting his "whole time to pushing the Townsend pension plan." Sacramento *Union*, Apr. 22, 1935. Needless to say, nothing came of these fanciful schemes.

70. Blackorby, pp. 219–25; Holtzman, *Townsend Movement*, pp. 170–78; Bennett, pp. 9–10, 14–15, 198–200.

71. Calif. [53], Presidential Primary Election, May 5, 1936, pp. 40–63; Cresap, p. 70; *EPIC News*, Mar. 9, Mar. 16, Apr. 20, 1936; McIntosh, pp. 358–59.

72. *EPIC News*, May 18, 1936.

73. *Ibid.*

74. *EPIC News*, June 8, Nov. 2, Nov. 30, Dec. 7, 1936, July 19, Sept. 27, 1937.

CHAPTER 4

1. For Townsend's life see Harris, p. 455, and Townsend's *Autobiography*, esp. pp. 2, 8, 25, 46–60, 74–97, 101–36. Two rather hostile descriptions of Townsend's early promotional ventures are U.S. [15], Vol. I, pp. 6–10; and Whiteman and Lewis, pp. 64–65.

2. Milne, p. 2.

3. *Modern Crusader*, Jan. 5, 1935.

4. Townsend, *Autobiography*, pp. 135–43. That the garbage can story is merely a myth is persuasively argued in Holtzman, "Townsend Movement" (diss.), pp. 63–66, and in the same author's book, *Townsend Movement*, pp. 32–35. A recent historical work that repeats this colorful fable is Schlesinger, pp. 29–30. Schlesinger's use of the story is surprising, since he cites Holtzman's dissertation as a source for his chapter "The Old Folks' Crusade."

5. See Barton's "How to Fix Everything."

6. McCord's plan was copyrighted on August 7, 1931. Holtzman, *Townsend Movement*, pp. 34–35. As Holtzman notes (p. 35), even the $200 pension and the compulsory-spending idea were hinted at in Mc-Cord's proposal.

7. *Ibid.*, p. 35.

8. Apr. 8, 1931, Mar. 21, Apr. 3, 1933. Furthermore, the Technocrats had proposed that citizens be required to spend government subsidies paid to them. McIntosh, p. 101.

9. Townsend, *Autobiography*, p. 138; Holtzman, *Townsend Movement*, pp. 35–40.

10. The pamphlet is reprinted in O'Byrne, p. 179. To make matters more complicated as well as more comical, these two distortions of history in effect canceled each other out, for whereas the first changed the $150 figure to $200 and left the sales tax untouched, the second replaced the sales tax by a gross income tax but returned to the original pension figure of $150 a month.

11. *National Townsend Weekly*, Apr. 13, 1936, p. 2.

12. *Modern Crusader*, Nov. 3, 1934; Sacramento *Union*, Apr. 21, Apr. 22, 1937; Sacramento *Bee*, May 13, 1940.

13. O'Byrne, p. 93.

14. See the indignant poem by James Jones entitled "Just Who?" for a striking articulation of this theme. *Modern Crusader*, Sept. 29, 1934. The psychological importance of the movement's ability to preserve or enhance "self-regard" is dealt with ably by Cantril, chap. 7.

15. Holtzman, *Townsend Movement*, p. 46.

16. Holtzman, "Townsend Movement" (diss.), pp. 278–79. In a politically atomized community like California the sense of political isolation was probably stronger than elsewhere and consequently the sense of participation provided by the Townsend clubs was probably stronger than elsewhere. Under these circumstances it is not surprising that one psychologist remarked, "Perhaps the greatest part of the popularity of Townsendism stemmed from a psychological rather than an economic need." George Lawton, "Psychological Guidance for Older Persons," in Cowdry (1942), p. 795.

17. Most of the ideas expressed here on Townsend's conservative-radical synthesis are taken from Holtzman, *Townsend Movement*, pp. 43–45.

18. Holtzman, "Townsend Movement" (diss.), pp. 43–61. On the pronounced Midwestern, middle-class, Protestant makeup of Townsend's following, see Bennett, pp. 167–69.

19. Townsend, *Autobiography*, pp. 168–70.

20. Townsend, for example, castigated the Roosevelt administration for "repudiating its solemn obligations to pay its bonds in gold." *Ibid.*, pp. 238–39. This was a curious criticism in view of the financial highjinks Townsend had advocated.

21. *Ibid.*, pp. 67–69. Townsend invariably concluded, however, for the

sake of consistency, that the plight of the poor in the modern industrial era was worse than the privations endured by the pioneers, thus making the Townsend pensions justifiable and necessary. *Ibid.*, pp. 7, 128–36, 220–25, 237.

22. Holtzman, "Townsend Movement" (diss.), pp. 119–20, 279–81.

23. For a bombastic example see Dorman, pp. 20–23.

24. *National Townsend Weekly*, Apr. 11, 1936. According to one unverified account, Townsend "once remarked to his friends that if the nation of today so lauded Lincoln who had freed a few million colored people from chattel slavery, what would the nation of tomorrow think of him (Townsend) who was freeing everybody from economic and debt slavery." Whiteman and Lewis, p. 266. For other efforts to rank Townsend with great American historical personages see *National Townsend Weekly*, Jan. 4 and Jan. 11, 1937.

25. Charles T. Murdock in *National Townsend Weekly*, Aug. 12, 1934, quoted in O'Byrne, pp. 80–81.

26. *Modern Crusader*, Oct. 17, 1934.

27. Nell Mandeville, "The Turn of the Road," in *ibid.*, Dec. 1, 1934.

28. Townsend, *Autobiography*, p. 20.

29. "And Jesus, walking by the sea of Galilee, saw two brethren, Simon called Peter, and Andrew his brother, casting a net into the sea; for they were fishers. And he saith unto them, Follow me and I will make you fishers of men. And they straightway left their nets and followed him." Matt. 4:18–20.

30. The best economic analysis of the plan is *The Townsend Crusade*. Less restrained but basically sound is Neuberger and Loe, chap. 10. See also "Agitation for Pension and Scrip Schemes," pp. 237–39. Good summaries of the plan's weaknesses can be found in Holtzman, *Townsend Movement*, pp. 108–10, and in Bennett, pp. 159–61.

31. San Francisco *Chronicle*, Jan. 12, 1936.

32. Letter from Marion P. Bush in *ibid.*, Jan. 30, 1936.

33. San Francisco *Chronicle*, Jan. 9, 1936, p. F-1. Furthermore, a later poll revealed that when people were asked to register mere approval or disapproval of the plan without mentioning the size of the pensions involved, as many as 35 per cent of the sample approved the plan. This survey also showed that the poor, and in particular those on relief, of whom California had a large number, were heavily in favor of the plan. Cantril, pp. 191–93; Holtzman, *Townsend Movement*, pp. 83–84.

34. Redlands *Daily Facts*, Apr. 2, 1936; Santa Rosa *Press-Democrat*, Oct. 14, 1934, Sept. 18, 1935. For editorials genuinely friendly to the plan see those by R. Beardsworth Curtis, Pasadena *Star-News*, May 9, 1934, and by Manchester Boddy, Los Angeles *Daily News*, Sept. 26, 1934, reprinted in *Modern Crusader*, Sept. 29, 1934. For hostile though restrained editorials from a town heavily populated with old people and Townsendites, see Santa Cruz *News*, Aug. 2, Sept. 1, Sept. 4, Sept. 6, Oct. 3, 1934.

35. Townsend, *Autobiography*, pp. 142–47; U.S. [15], Vol. I, pp. 10,

15–16; Mason, p. 37. On Clements see *ibid.* and Harris, p. 456. Clements claimed that he became convinced of the workability of the plan by reading economics in the Long Beach Public Library.

36. Harris, p. 456; U.S. [15], Vol. I, pp. 19, 121–22.

37. U.S. [15], Vol. I, pp. 121–26; Holtzman, *Townsend Movement*, pp. 66–67; Townsend, *Autobiography*, p. 22.

38. On the Los Angeles meetings see Neuberger and Loe, pp. 64–65. On those in San Diego see *ibid.*, p. 65, and Lake, p. 12.

39. Lake, pp. 13, 121–22; Leuchtenburg, p. 104.

40. Neuberger and Loe, p. 66.

41. U.S. [15], Vol. I, pp. 26–27, 31; O'Byrne, pp. 50–52; Neuberger and Loe, p. 67.

42. Mason, pp. 44–45; Harris, p. 456. The largest club on record was organized by "live wire" George Highley in Los Angeles. It had some 22,000 members. Later the organization voted to limit clubs to a maximum of 1,000 members. U.S. [15], Vol. I, pp. 42–43.

43. O'Byrne, p. 50; Holtzman, *Townsend Movement*, pp. 56–57; *Modern Crusader*, Dec. 1, 1934, p. 4. Townsend at one time spoke of building "Townsend centers" for the use of his clubs, "which are to be like Carnegie Libraries with additional social activities." *Townsend Crusade*, p. 10. Apparently these centers never materialized.

44. Townsend, *Autobiography*, pp. 149, 162; U.S. [15], Vol. I, pp. 161–62.

45. Townsend, *Autobiography*, p. 152. Townsend and Clements again used a "dummy" incorporator in this action. See U.S. [15], Vol. I, pp. 162–65.

46. McDonald claimed that Clements was able to begin publishing the *Weekly* only by stealing the *Crusader*'s subscription list, but this sensational charge was never proved. U.S. [15], Vol. I, pp. 162–63; *Modern Crusader*, Dec. 22, 1934, Jan. 5, 1935; Neuberger and Loe, pp. 112–13.

47. Whiteman and Lewis, p. 74; Townsend, *Autobiography*, p. 182; Holtzman, *Townsend Movement*, pp. 71–72.

48. Holtzman, "Townsend Movement" (diss.), p. 307.

49. "There was no need to convert the spectacular claims, the glitter, the bold assertions of economic assumptions as verities into sober and specific terms." *Ibid.*, pp. 61–62. See also Holtzman, *Townsend Movement*, pp. 35–46.

50. U.S. [15], Vol. I, pp. 3–211, 333–76. It might be said on Townsend's behalf that he got rid of Clements when some of Clements's more damaging actions and statements were disclosed, but it would be difficult to prove that Townsend was morally outraged by these disclosures rather than merely aware that Clements had become a political liability. Townsend, *Autobiography*, p. 153; *National Townsend Weekly*, Apr. 13, 1936. There is also evidence that Townsend's dismissal of Clements merely reflected the outcome of a power struggle between the two. O'Byrne, pp. 95–98.

51. Mason, p. 44; Whiteman and Lewis, pp. 82–84.

52. Whiteman and Lewis, pp. 82–84; U.S. [15], Vol. I, pp. 10, 109–12. Margett had been charged, but not convicted, of receiving and spending the earnings of a prostitute, and had also been indicted for grand larceny and bootlegging. Holtzman, *Townsend Movement*, p. 165.

53. Alsop and Kintner, pp. 5–7, 85–87, 89–90; *National Townsend Weekly*, Apr. 13, 1936; Townsend, *Autobiography*, p. 159. A look at any of Downey's books indicates that he had a fairly sophisticated understanding of the functioning of a modern economy. In *Why I Believe in the Townsend Plan* he made an intelligent, if not altogether successful, attempt to place the Townsend plan on sounder economic grounds.

54. U.S. [15], Vol. I, pp. 126–30.

55. O'Byrne, pp. 55–57.

56. Holtzman, "Townsend Movement" (diss.), p. 287. The name of the national organization was changed to Townsend National Recovery Plan, Inc., in 1936, and to Townsend Plan, Inc., in 1948. See also Holtzman, *Townsend Movement*, pp. 66–76.

57. *Modern Crusader*, Sept. 29, 1934; Santa Cruz *News*, Aug. 16, 1935.

58. O'Byrne, p. 71.

59. Holtzman, *Townsend Movement*, p. 79. For examples of Townsend's rather blasé attitudes about soliciting money from members see Sacramento *Union*, Apr. 22, 1937; Santa Cruz *News*, Sept. 10, 1937; and Townsend, *Autobiography*, p. 164.

60. Holtzman, *Townsend Movement*, pp. 71–72.

61. U.S. [15], Vol. I, pp. 180–87; Holtzman, *Townsend Movement*, p. 82.

62. U.S. [15], Vol. I, pp. 147, 659–61; Neuberger and Loe, pp. 139–45; Mason, pp. 39–40; Bennett, pp. 170–71.

63. Sacramento *Union*, May 17, 1935; Neuberger and Loe, pp. 146–47.

64. San Francisco *Chronicle*, May 24, 1935; *National Townsend Weekly*, June 24, 1935; Mason, pp. 39–40; Santa Cruz *News*, Sept. 23, 1935.

65. San Francisco *Chronicle*, Sept. 12, Sept. 13, Sept. 16, 1935; Whiteman and Lewis, p. 111; Neuberger and Loe, p. 152.

66. Santa Cruz *News*, Sept. 20, Sept. 21, Sept. 23, Sept. 24, Nov. 9, Nov. 11, 1935; San Francisco *Chronicle*, Sept. 22, Nov. 11, 1935.

67. San Francisco *Chronicle*, Apr. 8, 1936; O'Byrne, pp. 95–98. This uprising was probably as much a part of Clements's unsuccessful attempt to take over the movement and his eventual defeat and dismissal as it was a reform move by the rank and file.

68. O'Byrne, pp. 37–38; Sacramento *Union*, Jan. 19, Mar. 14, 1937.

69. San Francisco *Chronicle*, June 19, 1937; Holtzman, *Townsend Movement*, pp. 111, 113, 144.

70. O'Byrne, pp. 57–60.

71. There was an attempt to unite the Hudson and Daley groups, but nothing came of it. San Francisco *Chronicle*, Nov. 11, 1935.

72. Santa Cruz *News*, Sept. 23, Oct. 28, 1935; *National Townsend Weekly*, Oct. 21, 1935.

73. Of course, the Townsendites also intervened in California congres-

sional races and tried to influence the congressmen to vote for Townsend measures, but these were essentially national political affairs, and furthermore the Townsend efforts in this regard were extremely haphazard and ineffective. O'Byrne, pp. 133–34, 138–40, 150–53, 155; Holtzman, "Townsend Movement" (diss.), pp. 349–51, 364–65, 556; *Modern Crusader,* Nov. 3, Dec. 8, 1934; *National Townsend Weekly,* Aug. 31, Sept. 28, 1936, July 11, Oct. 31, 1938.

74. *Modern Crusader,* Sept. 29, 1934.

75. O'Byrne, p. 34; San Francisco *Chronicle,* Jan. 27, 1935; Lake, pp. 13, 127; *Modern Crusader,* Nov. 3, 1934.

76. *National Townsend Weekly,* Jan. 21, 1935.

77. Sacramento *Union,* Jan. 23, 1935.

78. *National Townsend Weekly,* Jan. 28, 1935; Assembly Joint Resolution No. 6, *Statutes of California,* 1935, chap. 30.

79. Sacramento *Union,* Mar. 5, 1935. Characteristically, Merriam had especially high praise for the plan's sales tax feature, "in which everyone would participate according to his means and buying power."

80. This episode is chronicled in the Sacramento *Union,* Mar. 8–12, 1935.

81. *Ibid.,* Mar. 13, 1935.

82. *Ibid.,* Mar. 20, 1935; O'Byrne, pp. 119–20. Olson's fellow EPIC legislator, Assemblyman Ellis Patterson, also opposed the resolution vociferously. Sacramento *Union,* Mar. 9, 1935.

83. O'Byrne, pp. 122–23; Sacramento *Union,* Mar. 14, Mar. 15, Mar. 19, 1935. Merriam said of his postponement tactic, "I'm just letting nature take its course." *Ibid.,* Mar. 14, 1935.

84. *Ibid.,* Mar. 15, Mar. 14, 1935.

85. *Ibid.,* Mar. 20, 1935; *Statutes of California,* 1935, chap. 57.

86. The resolution was twice reenacted by the legislature, once in 1936 and again in 1944, with the usual lack of response from Congress. San Francisco *Chronicle,* May 27, 1936; Holtzman, "Townsend Movement" (diss.), p. 566.

87. Although Merriam continued to cultivate the support of the Townsendites, his efforts did his career little good. He was not reelected governor in 1938, nor was he elected to any other office thereafter. Sacramento *Union,* Apr. 21, 1935; Santa Rosa *Press-Democrat,* July 18, 1935; *National Townsend Weekly,* Sept. 9, Nov. 25, 1935, July 4, 1938, Mar. 16, 1940.

88. Carlson, p. 306.

89. "Agitation for Pension and Scrip Schemes," p. 236; Calif. [9], p. 30; Mason, pp. 38–39; Townsend, *Autobiography,* pp. 165, 186.

90. There is some evidence that the controversy over the second McGroarty bill helped spark the Oakland and Santa Cruz defections from the movement. Whiteman and Lewis, p. 111; Neuberger and Loe, pp. 146–47.

91. "Because of the efforts of our national membership," said Townsend in 1943, "the aged people of this nation today are receiving millions

of dollars annually in the form of old-age pensions which they had never received before. This is the result of the individual work of our members carrying forward the message of security and thus making our nation pension-conscious." Townsend, *Autobiography*, p. 235. On the question of the influence of the Townsend plan on the passage of the Social Security Act, see Schlesinger, pp. 40–41; Francis Perkins, *The Roosevelt I Knew* (New York, 1940), pp. 278–79, 294; Witte, pp. 96, 103; and Altmeyer, pp. 9–10, 11, 13, 32, 37.

92. O'Byrne, p. 141.

93. U.S. [15], Vol. I, pp. 769–70. Townsend was later convicted of contempt by a federal court and sentenced to jail. President Roosevelt shrewdly pardoned him, however, thereby depriving him of his martyrdom. It is generally conceded by students of the plan that this committee, headed by Representative C. Jasper Bell of Missouri, subjected Townsend to some very rough and unfair treatment. O'Byrne, p. 141; Holtzman, *Townsend Movement*, pp. 161–66. Most California newspapers were much more critical of the committee's tactics than they were of Townsend in the affair. Long Beach *Press-Telegram*, Feb. 20, 1936, Feb. 25, 1937; San Francisco *Chronicle*, Feb. 22, 1938; Santa Cruz *News*, Mar. 9, May 12, 1936, Feb. 27, Apr. 13, 1937; Redlands *Daily Facts*, Feb. 16, 1938. The *National Townsend Weekly* was naturally outraged by the Bell Committee's actions. Mar. 30, Apr. 20, 1936, Mar. 14, 1938.

94. Mason, pp. 42–43; Holtzman, *Townsend Movement*, pp. 172–78; *National Townsend Weekly*, Apr. 13, Oct. 12, 1936; Bennett, pp. 138–44, 178–84.

95. Holtzman, "Townsend Movement" (diss.), pp. 381–87; O'Byrne, pp. 99, 116–18; San Francisco *Chronicle*, June 14, June 19, 1937, Feb. 3, 1939; Corson and McConnell, pp. 119–20.

96. Holtzman, "Townsend Movement" (diss.), pp. 350–51, 562–63; *National Townsend Weekly*, Apr. 10, June 23, July 7, 1939.

97. *National Townsend Weekly*, Oct. 3, 1938; Santa Rosa *Press-Democrat*, June 16, 1938; Holtzman, *Townsend Movement*, pp. 184–87.

98. The platform demonstrated clearly, too, that the Townsend movement harbored some pronounced elements of political conservatism. Besides advocating a national Townsend plan law, it favored protecting American goods from foreign competition, reducing the number of government agencies, stopping government competition with private enterprise, and including the public as a legitimate third party in all labor disputes. Holtzman, *Townsend Movement*, p. 184. As for the congressional elections, the Townsendites won little support, owing largely to their ineptitude. In their confusion they fielded candidates against friends as well as enemies. Some California congressmen, apparently resenting this treatment, then became opponents of the plan. *Ibid.*, pp. 185–86.

99. Calif. [53], Primary Election, 1938, General Election, 1938; *National Townsend Weekly*, Oct. 31, 1938; Holtzman, *Townsend Movement*, pp. 185–86; O'Byrne, pp. 146–48, 157–58. The party did support

the cross-filings on its ticket of state Senator Ralph Swing and candidate for United States Senator Sheridan Downey. Both were victorious, but in all probability would have won without Townsend's endorsement. O'Byrne, p. 146; Holtzman, *Townsend Movement*, p. 185.

100. Calif. [53], Primary Election, 1940, General Election, 1940, Primary Election, 1942, General Election, 1942; O'Byrne, pp. 147, 149, 157–58; Holtzman, *Townsend Movement*, p. 186. The party may have influenced some local elections but it never gave them any publicity except for the San Francisco mayoralty contest in 1939, in which it supported the loser. O'Byrne, pp. 149–50.

101. For my analysis of the failure of the Townsend Party, I have depended heavily on Holtzman, "Townsend Movement" (diss.), pp. 492–500.

102. It might be argued that the Townsend Party was more successful in the senatorial contest of 1938, in which it helped secure the supposedly sympathetic services of Senator Sheridan Downey. Downey's election, however, should probably be credited mainly to the support of another pension organization, the Ham and Eggs movement, and although he cultivated the continued support of the Townsendites, even to the extent of introducing a Townsend old-age pension bill in the Senate in 1940, his sincerity on the whole issue of the Townsend plan by this time was very doubtful. San Francisco *Chronicle*, July 15, 1939, Jan. 26, 1940; *National Townsend Weekly*, Aug. 25, 1939, Nov. 10, Apr. 20, 1940; Holtzman, "Townsend Movement" (diss.), pp. 400–401, 476–80.

103. O'Byrne, pp. 39, 70. The California section in the *Weekly* began in the Feb. 6, 1939, issue and ended with the Dec. 7, 1940, issue.

104. O'Byrne, p. 39; *National Townsend Weekly*, June 1, 1940; Sacramento *Bee*, Feb. 20, May 21, 1940.

105. O'Byrne, pp. 40–42; *National Townsend Weekly*, Dec. 1, Dec. 30, 1939, Jan. 27, Feb. 3, 1940.

106. *National Townsend Weekly*, May 4, 1940. The fate of this proposed amendment is chronicled in *ibid.*, May 18, June 8, June 22, July 20, 1940.

107. O'Byrne, pp. 43, 160–61.

108. Letter from John C. Cuneo to California State Advisory Board, no date. Quoted in Messinger, p. 5.

109. Holtzman, "Townsend Movement" (diss.), pp. 505, 507, 515; O'Byrne, pp. 70, 121–23, 125, 127.

110. See Messinger.

CHAPTER 5

1. Whiteman and Lewis, p. 219. The Republican Party in California was undergoing moderate liberalization at this time. Merriam was not an enthusiastic exponent of this process, but he at least accepted it and gave the appearance of promoting it. Cresap, pp. 27–28.

2. Sacramento *Union*, Jan. 9, 1935.

3. *Ibid.*, Jan. 23, Mar. 3, 1935.

4. Burke, pp. 8–9.

5. Sacramento *Union,* Jan. 15, Apr. 11, Apr. 12, May 5, May 27, May 28, 1935; Walker and Cave, p. 191. Demands for severance taxes were defeated, as they have been to this day—a tribute to the power of the oil lobby. Hyink et al., p. 218. Another Merriam victory was the passage of the Wright Act, which limited department and county budgets to a maximum of 105 per cent of the preceding year's budget. This was a source of comfort to propertied folk fearful of increased county levies and heavier budget requests by state administrators. Sacramento *Union,* June 4, 1935.

6. Sacramento *Union,* Jan. 16, Apr. 12, 1937.

7. Sacramento *Bee,* Mar. 7, 1938; Santa Rosa *Press-Democrat,* Dec. 17, 1937.

8. Sacramento *Union,* May 16, 1935, Apr. 20, 1937.

9. Sacramento *Union,* Jan. 15, Jan. 19, Mar. 21, Apr. 2, Apr. 8, Apr. 20, Apr. 25, June 4, 1935.

10. Peirce, p. 87; Calif. [24], July 1938–June 1940, p. 27. By December 1938 California was paying pensions to some 26.3 per cent of her 65-and-over population, whereas the nation at large was paying pensions to 21.8 per cent. California was outdone in this regard by Colorado and Oklahoma, which paid pensions to 46.1 and 54.5 per cent of their respective aged populations. Kulp, p. 72.

11. Calif. [5], p. 1988. Beginning in 1936, however, the federal government paid large portions of these pensions under the Social Security Act.

12. Peirce, pp. 89–90; U.S. [13], p. 25. The latter source lists California as having the highest individual pensions in the nation, although it gives a slightly higher pension figure for December 1938 ($32.97) than does the former source ($32.43). The latter figure is also given in Calif. [24], July 1938–June 1940, p. 27. As usual, the size of pensions continued to vary considerably from county to county.

13. *California Statutes,* 1935, chap. 1, Assembly Joint Resolution no. 1.

14. Calif. [40], *AB,* 1935, AB 49; Calif. [42], *JA,* 51st sess., 1935, pp. 46, 5111–12; Sacramento *Union,* Jan. 10, 1935, p. 12. At least four similar bills introduced at about the same time were immediately stifled in committee. Calif. [42], *JA,* 51st sess., 1935, pp. 38, 126, 150, 5111–12.

15. Witte, pp. 79–81.

16. Calif. [46], *SB,* 1935, SB 12, SB 942; Calif. [43], *JS,* 51st sess., 1935, pp. 44, 370, 1424–25, 1439–41, 1527, 1916, 2161, 2180, 2214, 2222, 2230–31, 2341, 2532–33, 2693, 2694, 2717–18, 3009, 3320, 3332–33; Calif. [42], *JA,* 51st sess., 1935, pp. 4570, 5113. Both of these bills also provided for lowering the age limit to 65 and reducing other requirements for eligibility.

17. Swing's argument is to be found in the Sacramento *Union,* May 22 and June 5, 1935.

18. Sacramento *Union,* June 5, 1935.

19. *Ibid.* Olson's impassioned oratory here was not all poetic license, as the Philbrick report on California lobbying would soon reveal. It may have hit home to Senator Swing at the time, since the Philbrick report

showed him to be closely associated with various powerful lobbies. Philbrick, pp. 50–54; see also Cresap, p. 107.

20. Sacramento *Union*, June 5, 1935; Calif. [46], *SB*, 1935, SB 12; Calif. [43], *JS*, 51st sess., 1935, p. 2694.

21. Calif. [43], *JS*, 51st sess., 1935, pp. 3009, 3320; Calif. [42], *JA*, 51st sess., 1935, pp. 4570, 5113.

22. Calif. [40], *AB*, 1935, AB 767; Calif. [42], *JA*, 51st sess., 1935, pp. 317, 1779, 1809–10, 2046, 2533, 2556–57, 3213, 3607, 4082, 4212, 4244, 4250, 4252, 4253, 4254, 4255–56, 4258, 4259, 4555, 4657, 4999, 5124; Calif. [43], *JS*, 51st sess., 1935, pp. 2778, 2910, 2918, 3004–5, 3007, 3008, 3146; *California Statutes*, 1935, chap. 633. One of these amendments was a typically unsuccessful attempt by Olson to raise the pension to $50 a month. *JS*. pp. 3004–5, 3007.

23. The major changes in the law are conveniently summarized in Calif. [24], July 1934–June 1936, pp. 22–23. See also Redlands *Daily Facts*, Aug. 19, 1935.

24. These reactions were recorded in the Sacramento *Union*, June 15, 1935.

25. *Ibid.* See also Santa Cruz *News*, Aug. 6, 1935.

26. San Francisco *Chronicle*, May 7, 1936; Redlands *Daily Facts*, Feb. 5, 1935. In 1939 a California judge denied the naturalization petition of an alien on the ground that his only motivation for becoming a citizen was to draw a pension. Los Angeles *Times*, Dec. 19, 1939.

27. Sacramento *Union*, June 15, 1935.

28. San Francisco *Chronicle*, May 5, May 7, 1936; Santa Cruz *News*, Mar. 26, 1936.

29. Santa Cruz *News*, Dec. 19, 1935.

30. San Francisco *Chronicle*, Jan. 15, 1936. Brennan was chairman of the Assembly Social Welfare Committee. The investigation was urged by the FOE.

31. *Ibid.*, Jan. 30, 1936. For some corroboration of the grocery-order charge, see *ibid.*, Aug. 21, 1936.

32. *Ibid.*, Jan. 21, Jan. 30, 1936.

33. Long Beach *Press-Telegram*, Feb. 5, 1936; San Francisco *Chronicle*, May 28, 1936.

34. *California Statutes*, 1937, chap. 7; Calif. [24], July 1934–June 1936, pp. 24–25; San Francisco *Chronicle*, May 27, 1936. The new provision on property ownership declared that the home of an aged person should no longer be considered the home of the person's spouse if the two were separated and maintaining separate residences, even though they may not have been divorced.

35. Pasadena *Star-News*, Aug. 21, 1936; Peirce, pp. 86–89; Calif. [24], July 1934–June 1936, bet. pp. 20–21, and July 1936–June 1938, p. 20. Merriam's remark was quoted in the San Francisco *Chronicle*, May 28, 1936.

36. Calif. [5], p. 1988.

37. Sacramento *Union*, Jan. 16, 1937; San Francisco *Chronicle*, Feb.

4, 1937; Calif. [5], p. 1988. The state and local share of the expenditures for old-age pensions rose from $7.2 million in fiscal 1935–36 to $12.8 million in fiscal 1936–37, to $21.6 million in fiscal 1937–38. *Ibid.*

38. Calif. [5], p. 2004.

39. Calif. [40], *AB*, 1937, AB 524; Calif. [42], *JA*, 52d sess., 1937, pp. 244, 1311–13, 2644–45, 3126–27, 3292, 3869; Calif. [43], *JS*, 52d sess., 1937, pp. 2369, 2565, 2585–86, 2632, 2671; *California Statutes*, 1937, chap. 392.

40. Fitzgerald, p. 6.

41. Calif. [29], Jan. 1937, p. 10, and Mar. 1937, p. 19.

42. Calif. [40], *AB*, 1937, AB 534; Calif. [42], *JA*, 52d sess., 1937, p. 245.

43. California State Chamber of Commerce, p. 9; Sacramento *Union*, Jan. 16, May 12, 1937; Santa Rosa *Press-Democrat*, Jan. 16, 1937; Redlands *Daily Facts*, Feb. 8, Mar. 11, June 3, 1937; Calif. [24], July 1936–June 1938, p. 14.

44. *EPIC News*, Mar. 29, Apr. 12, Apr. 19, May 10, 1937; Redlands *Daily Facts*, Feb. 8, 1937, Long Beach *Press-Telegram*, Jan. 6, 1937. Colorado lowered its pension age to 60 and raised its maximum monthly payment to $45. This provision later resulted in serious financial difficulties, however, and Colorado's experience probably provided more ammunition for the opponents than for the advocates of increased pensions. "Agitation for Pension and Scrip Schemes," pp. 233–36; Pasadena *Star-News*, Dec. 28, 1939.

45. Calif. [42], *JA*, 52d sess., 1937, pp. 245, 1061, 1134, 1252, 2637, 2682, 2735, 2760–61, 3208, 3237, 3338; Calif. [40], *AB*, 1937, AB 2919; *California Statutes*, 1937, chaps. 49, 369.

46. San Francisco *Chronicle*, June 14, 1937; Pasadena *Star-News*, July 22, 1937. During a discussion of this bill in which it was alleged, with gross exaggeration, that the proposal would increase financial burdens on the counties by $20 million a year, Hornblower candidly declared, "The heat's been turned on this measure. . . . I'm frank to say I don't know where the counties are going to get $20,000,000 a year more." Sacramento *Union*, Mar. 13, 1937.

47. Calif. [40], *AB*, 1937, AB 1; Calif. [42], 52d sess., 1937, pp. 34, 1060, 1103–5, 1350, 2201, 2214–15, 2643, 3545, 3572–78, 3868; Calif. [43], *JS*, 52d sess., 1937, pp. 2369, 2565, 2579–83, 2844–45, 2899, 2955, 3064; *California Statutes*, 1937, chap. 405.

48. Calif. [42], *JA*, 52d sess., 1937, p. 3868; Sacramento *Union*, Apr. 7, 1937, p. 13.

49. The main provisions of this act (*California Statutes*, 1937, chap. 405) are summarized in Peirce, p. 3. See also Calif. [5], p. 1964; Calif. [24], July 1936–June 1938, pp. 5, 8–11, 14–16, and July 1938–June 1940, pp. 8, 9.

50. For a perceptive analysis of the phenomenon of "slight privilege" among the older age groups, see Pinner et al., pp. 91–107, 267–68.

51. Bond et al., pp. 315–16.

52. Pensioners whose property was partly encumbered by private mortgages were also helped by the repeal of the lien provision, since under

the old system a person who held a mortgage on a pensioner's property was well-advised to foreclose to protect his investment. An earlier bill sponsored by Senator John Phillips that permitted county boards to release liens in order to prevent such foreclosures was given an emergency rating and enacted into law early in the 1937 session. This discretionary provision was, of course, superseded by the Hornblower Act of 1937, but it was useful to the otherwise conservative Senator Phillips in demonstrating his concern for the welfare of his aged constituents, and he exploited it considerably. John Phillips, *Inside California*, p. 150; Calif. [46], *SB*, 1937, SB 159; Calif. [43], *JS*, 52d sess., 1937, pp. 165, 234, 315, 346, 433; *California Statutes*, 1937, chap. 4.

53. Bond et al., p. 315.

54. Calif. [24], 1927–28, pp. 182–83; Bond et al., pp. 320–22.

55. Pasadena *Star-News*, June 18, Aug. 26, 1937. The August 26 editorial went on to justify the entire pension system in terms that amounted to a repetition of the typical arguments used by pension spokesmen. This may indicate that the old-age political movement was beginning to have some success in influencing public opinion.

56. *Ibid.*, Aug. 12, 1937. These estimates were actually lower than the increased coverage and cost of pensions in the county, for during the fiscal year 1937–38 the number of pensioners in Los Angeles County increased by more than 17,000, and the cost of pensions by almost $6 million. In August 1937 the Los Angeles County Superintendent of Charities said that new pension applications were being filed at an unprecedented rate (more than 500 applications on the first day of filing) and estimated that by January 1, 1938, the county would have an all-time high of 35,000 pensioners. As it turned out, the county had 36,364 by that date. Calif. [24], July 1936–June 1938, pp. 22–25; San Francisco *Chronicle*, Aug. 21, 1937.

57. Pasadena *Star-News*, Dec. 30, 1937.

58. San Francisco *Chronicle*, Jan. 17, 1938.

59. *Lake County Bee*, Jan. 6, 1938; Santa Rosa *Press-Democrat*, Dec. 18, 1937.

60. Sacramento *Bee*, Mar. 8, 1938.

61. *Ibid.*, Mar, 7, 1938. Patterson had introduced a similar bill in the 1937 session. *EPIC News*, Mar. 29, 1937.

62. *EPIC News*, Jan. 3, 1938; Sacramento *Bee*, Mar. 7, Mar. 14, 1938.

63. Santa Rosa *Press-Democrat*, Dec. 18, Dec. 22, 1937.

64. Sacramento *Bee*, Mar. 7, Mar. 8, 1938; Calif. [42], *JA*, 52d sess., 1938, pp. 7, 30, 31, 180; Calif. [43], *JS*, 52d sess., 1938, pp. 25, 54, 75, 179.

65. Sacramento *Bee*, Mar. 12, 1938.

66. *Ibid.*, Mar. 8, Mar. 9, 1938; Santa Cruz News, Mar. 10, 1938.

67. Calif. [43], *JS*, 52d sess., 1938, pp. 106, 120, 140, 162, 180; Calif. [42], *JA*, 52d sess., 1938, pp. 159–60; *California Statutes*, 1938, pp. 63–64.

68. Santa Cruz *News*, May 2, 1938; Pasadena *Star-News*, May 30, Aug. 31, 1938; *Lake County Bee*, June 16, 1938.

69. Calif. [24], July 1936–June 1938, p. 20, and July 1938–June 1940, p. 27.

70. Roseman, pp. 55–56; U.S. [13], p. 43; Glane, pp. 141–42.

71. For the director's story see the San Francisco *Chronicle*, Dec. 12, 1937.

72. *County of Los Angeles v. Jessup*, in *California Reports*, 2d ser., Vol. II (1938), pp. 273–83; Calif. [24], July 1936–June 1938, p. 16. The court reasoned that the law was invalid because it made a gift of "public money or thing of value" in violation of the California Constitution, it violated vested rights contrary to common law, and it fell afoul of the contract impairment clause of the United States Constitution. On each count, especially the last, the court's reasoning seems specious, and the decision was later reversed. See *County of Alameda v. Janssen*, in *California Reports*, 2d ser., Vol. XVI (1940–41), pp. 276–85.

CHAPTER 6

1. *EPIC News*, Dec. 27, 1937; Santa Cruz *News*, Sept. 23, 1937; Santa Rosa *Press-Democrat*, Aug. 12, 1938; Calif. [44], pp. 58–59; "Agitation for Pension and Scrip Schemes," p. 229.

2. Moore, pp. 16–17. The Moores' book, though highly partisan, has generally proved to be correct in its facts wherever I have been able to check them.

3. For Noble's brief career with EPIC, see *ibid.*, pp. 18–22.

4. *National Townsend Weekly*, Sept. 28, 1936.

5. Moore, p. 25; Fisher.

6. Fisher, "Stamped Scrip Plan," p. 164, and *Stamp Scrip*, pp. 48, 66–75.

7. Fisher, *Stamp Scrip*, pp. 17–44. Interestingly enough, two of the few places Fisher cited as having tried the scheme without success were the California towns of Merced and Anaheim. "In both places the plan had to be abandoned: in Merced for lack of enthusiasm; in Anaheim because of substantial loss." *Ibid.*, p. 36. For a further discussion of the Anaheim experience, see San Francisco *Chronicle*, Nov. 6, 1938. Redlands, California, also tried the scrip idea briefly in 1932, and apparently with some success. Redlands *Daily Facts*, Feb. 8, 1932. Whiteman and Lewis (p. 167) declared that such schemes failed in the state because "California was and still is to a certain extent, the land of gold, and has always leaned toward 'hard money.'" For another discussion of the various local scrip and currency schemes launched in America during the Depression, see Arthur Holch, "When Rubber Checks Didn't Bounce," *American Heritage*, XII (June 1961), 58–59.

8. Fisher, *Stamp Scrip*, pp. 53–75.

9. Fisher, "Stamped Scrip Plan," p. 164.

10. Fisher, *Stamp Scrip*, p. 67.

11. *Ibid.*, pp. 49–52.

12. Moore, p. 24; Sacramento *Union*, Apr. 13, 1937; O'Byrne, pp. 3–4. The EPIC organization had advocated both the issuance of scrip, though not of the stamp type, and increased pensions, but did not link the two. *EPIC News*, June 4, 1934.

13. Moore, pp. 24–25.

14. *Ibid.*, pp. 27–33. The statement that Willis Allen was formerly a

cheerleader is also in Boone, p. 31. A reference to Allen's career as a hair-tonic promoter can also be found in McWilliams, "Pension Politics," p. 321.

15. Moore, pp. 32–33.

16. *Ibid.*, pp. 33–36. The scandals of the Shaw administration became highly publicized, and Mayor Shaw was recalled by popular vote in 1938 for corruption in office. Nadeau, pp. 259–63; Crouch et al., pp. 124–25.

17. Moore, pp. 36–38.

18. This account of the takeover of Noble's organization comes from Moore, pp. 39–43, and McWilliams, "Ham and Eggs," p. 331.

19. Moore, pp. 43, 98–99. The Moores (p. 29) also cite a rumor that Lawrence Allen was a "diligent student of *Mein Kampf*" and sought to run the organization according to its principles. See also McWilliams, *Southern California Country*, pp. 307–8.

20. Chinn, pp. 41–43; Sinclair, *I, Candidate*, p. 38; Moore, p. 43.

21. Moore, pp. 48–49, 62; *EPIC News*, Nov. 11, 1935; Holtzman, "Townsend Movement" (diss.), p. 515. Another version of the origin of "Ham and Eggs" is that a speaker once promised his listeners that the movement would soon become as well-known to the California voter as ham and eggs. Cleland, p. 232.

22. Moore, pp. 58–62.

23. The information about Owens in this paragraph is taken from Moore, pp. 49–57, 99; Canterbury; and Boone. The quotations from Owens are in Boone, p. 30.

24. These events are chronicled in Moore, pp. 64–66.

25. Calif. [52], Propositions for Nov. 8, 1938, Election, Pt. II, Appendix, pp. 56–63.

26. Fisher's various criticisms of Ham and Eggs can be found in the San Diego *Sun*, Aug. 24, 1938; in "Agitation for Pension and Scrip Schemes," pp. 232–33; in the Pasadena *Star-News*, Oct. 6, 1938; and in a campaign brochure by the California Teachers Association, "Why You Should Vote No on Number 20, Single Tax and Vote No on Number 25, $30 Every Thursday," pp. 13–14, in the Bancroft Library Collection of Campaign Literature from the California Election of 1938.

27. Fisher estimated that the Ham and Eggs plan would necessitate the issuance of about $1.7 billion in warrants per year, whereas the average amount of currency and coin circulating in California was about $312 million per year. Fisher also asserted that stamp scrip could be made to work on the local level by securing adequate pledges of acceptance from banks and businesses, and on the national level by simply declaring the scrip to be legal tender. A state government, however, could use neither method.

28. For other trenchant criticisms of the plan see "Agitation for Pension and Scrip Schemes," pp. 231–32; "Hot Money for Californians"; Hamilton; and "$30 Every Thursday," pp. 300–301, 311–13.

29. *National Ham and Eggs*, Dec. 24, Dec. 31, 1938, Jan. 14, Jan. 28, Feb. 4, Mar. 18, 1939. This publication was the organization's weekly newspaper. It began publication on December 3, 1938.

30. Moore, pp. 68, 76–77, 111–12; McWilliams, "Ham and Eggs," p. 331.

31. Pinner et al., p. 6; Moore, p. 72; Canterbury, p. 409.

32. San Francisco *Chronicle*, Dec. 18, 1938, Oct. 6, 1939; *National Ham and Eggs*, Oct. 14, Dec. 23, 1939.

33. Boone, p. 31; Hamilton, p. 36.

34. *National Ham and Eggs*, Dec. 31, 1938, Oct. 14, 1939. The figure of over a million supporters was probably based on the fact that this many affirmative votes had been cast for the Ham and Eggs amendment in the 1938 election.

35. Almost every issue of *National Ham and Eggs* carried news of such meetings. A more sober account can be found in Canterbury, p. 408.

36. The newspaper article referred to in this paragraph is a United Press story from San Diego, Oct. 11, 1938, reprinted in the Santa Rosa *Press-Democrat*, Oct. 12, 1938. Closely related to the blind faith exhibited by the movement's followers was the repeated appeal by Ham and Eggs advocates to their skeptical opponents to withhold judgment on the plan, vote for it, and give it a "fair trial." Hamilton, p. 13.

37. My account of the Price incident is taken from Moore, pp. 63–64; McWilliams, *Southern California Country*, p. 306; Downey, *Pensions or Penury?*, pp. 26–27; and Alsop and Kintner, pp. 6–7. The quotation from Downey's oration is taken from *ibid.* The Ham and Eggers were not the first to exploit a suicide incident; they were only the most blatant. The passage of California's first old-age pension law in 1929 was probably facilitated by a similar incident. Putnam, "Influence of the Older Age Groups," p. 130. Likewise, the EPIC organization sought to exploit the "Andrew Black" suicide episode. *EPIC News*, Feb. 1, 1937.

38. Hamilton, p. 12; Moore, p. 77.

39. Pinner et al., pp. 6–7.

40. Campaign leaflets for Legg, Neblett, and Murphy, in Bancroft Library Collection of Campaign Literature from the California Election of 1938; Burke, pp. 14, 28; Santa Rosa *Press-Democrat*, Aug. 21, 1938. Murphy signed the opposition argument to Ham and Eggs in the voters' pamphlet in 1938. Calif. [52], Propositions for Nov. 8, 1938, Election, Pt. I, p. 48.

41. Burke, p. 16; Moore, pp. 83–84. According to the Moores it was Sherman Bainbridge who insisted that the Ham and Eggs organization refrain from endorsing a primary candidate and give Olson a fair chance. See also Kenny, p. 119.

42. Burke, pp. 12, 16–17; Olson campaign leaflets in Bancroft Library Collection of Campaign Literature from the California Election of 1938. The telegrams were later printed verbatim in *National Ham and Eggs*, July 8, 1939.

43. Calif. [53], Primary Election, Aug. 30, 1938, p. 21; Burke, p. 21; Alsop and Kintner, p. 87; "Agitation for Pension and Scrip Schemes," p. 227.

44. Calif. [53], Primary Election, Aug. 30, 1938, pp. 8–11. Patterson later asserted that unlike Downey, neither he nor Olson explicitly en-

dorsed the Ham and Eggs proposal, but his memory seems shaky on this point. Patterson, pp. 210–11.

45. Some of the more effective if unsubtle Ham and Eggs literature issued at this time was a pamphlet entitled "Life Begins at Fifty with $30 a Week for Life" and a leaflet made to look like a check issued by "Retirement Life Payments," dated November 8 (Election Day), and saying "Pay to the Order of You and Every California Citizen over Fifty, Thirty Dollars a Week for Life." Bancroft Library Collection of Campaign Literature from the California Election of 1938.

46. Canterbury, p. 409; Santa Rosa *Press-Democrat*, Sept. 23, 1938.

47. Long Beach *Press-Telegram*, Sept. 16, Oct. 31, 1938; Santa Rosa *Press-Democrat*, Oct. 22, 1938; Pasadena *Star-News*, Oct. 24, 1938. Attorney General U. S. Webb's opinion applied only to insurance companies, which he said could not handle the warrants without violating the state's rebate laws.

48. Bancroft Library Collection of Campaign Literature from the California Election of 1938; Los Angeles *Evening Herald-Express*, Nov. 4, 1938.

49. Santa Cruz *News*, Oct. 4, 1938.

50. San Francisco *Chronicle*, Aug. 13, 1938; *National Townsend Weekly*, Aug. 15, 1938; O'Byrne, pp. 159–60.

51. Moore, pp. 114–15, 119–20.

52. Roosevelt, who had swallowed his pride over Downey's defeat of McAdoo, willingly endorsed Downey for the party's sake, but continued to oppose Ham and Eggs. Patterson, p. 211; Burke, p. 28; Long Beach *Press-Telegram*, Oct. 5, 1938; Los Angeles *Evening Herald-Express*, Nov. 4, 1938. The old-time progressive Marshall Stimson opposed Downey because of the Ham and Eggs issue; see the typescript of his radio address on behalf of Bancroft, Nov. 7, 1938, in the Stimson Papers, and see also Bancroft, pp. 425–26, 452.

53. Burke, p. 24.

54. *Ibid.*, pp. 25–28; Santa Rosa *Press-Democrat*, Oct. 16, 1938; Long Beach *Press-Telegram*, Oct. 28, 1938.

55. Moore, pp. 92, 116, 122–23; Burke, p. 29; Santa Rosa *Press-Democrat*, Sept. 8, 1938. Bancroft Library Collection of Campaign Literature from the California Election of 1938. In this campaign Merriam continued to advocate the Townsend plan as a desirable alternative to Ham and Eggs. *National Townsend Weekly*, Sept. 26, 1938.

56. Calif. [53], Primary Election, Aug. 30, 1938, p. 7.

57. *The Noble News*, Oct. 22, 1938. This was a campaign newspaper of Noble's; it can be found in the California State Library Collection of Pension Plan Literature, Sacramento.

58. San Francisco *Chronicle*, Oct. 9, 1938; Los Angeles *Times*, Nov. 15, 1938; Los Angeles *Evening Herald-Express*, Nov. 15, 1938.

59. Moore, pp. 75–76, 85–89. According to the Moores, the Allens supported the Shaw administration only because they had been forced to do so by Kynette. The fact that the Allens had supported Shaw may have

been one reason why the new reform mayor, Fletcher Bowron, condemned the Ham and Eggs initiative in the November election. Los Angeles *Evening Herald-Express*, Nov. 3, 1938. See also Nadeau, pp. 260–62; Crouch et al., pp. 124–25. On Kynette's arrest and conviction, see Kenny, p. 112.

60. Moore, pp. 108–9; San Francisco *Chronicle*, Nov. 3, 1939; Los Angeles *Evening Herald-Express*, Nov. 2, Nov. 3, 1938; Los Angeles *Daily Journal*, Nov. 3, 1938; Los Angeles *Times*, Nov. 3, 1938; *Kynette v. California Pension Plan et al.*, Superior Court, Los Angeles County, Calif., file no. 433470. The forgery complaint brought by Berger was apparently dismissed when Willis Allen testified that he had signed Berger's name to the receipt with Berger's knowledge. Los Angeles *Evening Herald-Express*, Nov. 16, Nov. 17, 1938; Los Angeles *Times*, Nov. 17, 1938. A check of the records of the Los Angeles County Superior Court showed no record of a suit filed by Berger on this complaint.

61. The events described in this paragraph are discussed in Moore, pp. 113, 116–17.

62. Calif. [53], General Election, Nov. 8, 1938, p. 44.

63. Burke, p. 107; Moore, p. 133.

64. *National Ham and Eggs*, Dec. 3, 1938.

65. *Ibid.*, Feb. 4, 1939, Jan. 20, 1940; Burke, p. 107; Moore, pp. 131–54; San Francisco *Chronicle*, Feb. 12, 1939.

66. McWilliams, "Pension Politics," p. 320; Chinn, p. 68; Pinner et al., pp. 23–34. The last source contains the best account of McLain's early political activities.

67. *National Ham and Eggs*, Dec. 10, 1938; Pinner et al., p. 35.

68. Moore, pp. 157–58. A typical organization chart appears in *National Ham and Eggs*, Sept. 2, 1939, pp. 12–13. Under McLain's system the organization claimed to become national and even worldwide, with members not only in all 48 states but in several United States territories and foreign countries. *Ibid.*, Apr. 8, 1939.

69. *National Ham and Eggs*, Apr. 8, May 13, May 27, 1939; Moore, p. 183.

70. Copies and explanations of the proposal can be found in Calif. [52], Propositions for Nov. 7, 1939, Election, pp. 2–14; *National Ham and Eggs*, Dec. 24, 1938, Mar. 4, 1939; and Sacramento *Bee*, Jan. 16, 1939. Excellent criticisms of it can be found in "Threat of Pension Pressure Groups," pp. 1–7; Knepper; Moore, pp. 169–71; and Burke, p. 111.

71. *National Ham and Eggs*, Jan. 14, 1939.

72. Compare with Townsend's similar outpourings, p. 56 above, and a more recent effort by California's later pension messiah, George McLain, in *Senior Citizens Sentinel*, Feb. 1964.

73. On the average there were between 80 and 120 meetings a week. *National Ham and Eggs*, Feb. 4, Mar. 4, Apr. 8, May 6, June 10, July 8, Aug. 5, Sept. 9, 1939. For evidence of labor support see *ibid.*, Feb. 11, Mar. 25, May 6, June 10, 1939. For evidence of small-business support see *ibid.*, Mar. 11, Apr. 1, 1939.

74. Knepper, p. 64.

75. Moore, pp. 158–60; *National Ham and Eggs*, Apr. 15, 1939.

76. *National Ham and Eggs*, Dec. 17, 1938.

77. Examples of such editorials can be found in *ibid.*, Jan. 7, Jan. 28, 1939.

78. *The Noble News*, Dec. 19, 1938, Jan. 2, 1939, in the California State Library Collection of Pension Plan Literature, Sacramento, Sacramento *Bee*, Jan. 2, 1939; Santa Rosa *Press-Democrat*, Jan. 5, 1939. The juggling of the $25 and $30 figures shows that Noble was still trying to identify his movement with Ham and Eggs and to claim, in fact, that he had founded Ham and Eggs. The last placard is a reference to Roosevelt's denunciation of "short cuts to utopia."

79. Sacramento *Bee*, Jan. 3, 1939.

80. *National Ham and Eggs*, Dec. 31, 1938.

81. Sacramento *Bee*, May 1, 1939; Santa Rosa *Press-Democrat*, Apr. 25, 1939; *National Ham and Eggs*, Feb. 11, Apr. 29, May 6, 1939.

82. *National Ham and Eggs*, May 20, 1939.

83. *Ibid.*, May 27, 1939; Sacramento *Bee*, May 19, 1939; San Francisco *Chronicle*, May 18, 1939. The Allens claimed that a total of 1,103,222 signed petitions had been secured. This figure is probably fairly accurate.

84. *National Ham and Eggs*, May 27, 1939; San Francisco *Chronicle*, May 18, May 21, 1939, "This World" section; Sacramento *Bee*, May 18, May 19, 1939.

85. Sacramento *Bee*, May 19, 1939.

86. *National Ham and Eggs*, May 27, 1939.

87. *Ibid.*, May 20, 1939.

88. Santa Cruz *News*, Oct. 30, 1939.

89. *National Ham and Eggs*, June 10, Sept. 23, 1939. For denials of this charge see *Calaveras Prospect*, Aug. 12, 1939, and Redlands *Daily Facts*, Aug. 31, 1939.

90. A few examples of the sustained newspaper attack can be found in San Francisco *Chronicle*, Aug. 18, 1939; Long Beach *Press-Telegram*, Oct. 22, 1939; Pasadena *Star-News*, Oct. 5, 1939; Bakersfield *Californian*, Oct. 24, 1939; Santa Cruz *News*, Nov. 3, Nov. 6, 1939; *Calaveras Prospect*, Nov. 4, 1939.

91. Moore, p. 185. Obviously this speech bore little resemblance to Fisher's program, since Fisher proposed to work in close cooperation with bankers rather than to utterly alienate and antagonize them.

92. San Francisco *Chronicle*, July 22, Aug. 18, 1939; Pasadena *Star-News*, Nov. 3, 1939; Cleland, pp. 237–38; form letter in Stimson Papers dated Oct. 5, 1939; pamphlet of Southern California Citizens Against 30-Thursday, in Old-Age Pension Agitation Collection, Dept. of Special Collections, Univ. of Calif., Los Angeles, Library.

93. The curious opposition from labor came about because of a probably groundless fear that a minor section of the proposed act prohibiting the willful destruction of agricultural crops would jeopardize labor's right to picket farms and canneries. *National Ham and Eggs*, Sept. 23,

Oct. 7, Oct. 14, 1939; San Francisco *Chronicle*, Oct. 6, 1939. For the opposition of state employees and schoolteachers, see *ibid.*, July 7, 1939; Bakersfield *Californian*, Sept. 7, 1939; and *National Ham and Eggs*, Dec. 10, 1938. For the opposition of other pension leaders, see Cleland, p. 237; *National Townsend Weekly*, Nov. 17, 1939; Chinn, p. 160; and *The Noble News*, Jan. 2, 1939. Among those who brought suits against Ham and Eggs were several clerical employees who charged that they had been paid wages below those allowed by the state minimum-wage law; two former members of the organization's board of directors who claimed they had been illegally deprived of their positions; and an old lady who claimed she had been slapped in the face by Lawrence Allen. Only the last suit was lost by Ham and Eggs. San Francisco *Chronicle*, Apr. 16, June 4, Nov. 17, 1939; *National Ham and Eggs*, Dec. 2, 1939; Moore, pp. 123–24.

94. Sacramento *Bee*, May 23, 1939; Knepper, p. 58; Burke, p. 108.

95. *National Ham and Eggs*, June 3, June 17, June 24, July 1, 1939.

96. Burke, p. 109; Pasadena *Star-News*, July 7, 1939.

97. *National Ham and Eggs*, July 8, 1939.

98. *Ibid.*, July 8, July 22, Aug. 12, 1939.

99. Pasadena *Star-News*, July 7, 1939; San Francisco *Chronicle*, July 9, 1939, "This World" section; Burke, p. 109.

100. Burke, p. 110; *National Ham and Eggs*, Aug. 19, Aug. 26, 1939.

101. Santa Cruz *News*, Oct. 16, 1939; *National Ham and Eggs*, Apr. 8, Oct. 14, Oct. 21, 1939.

102. San Francisco *Chronicle*, Oct. 6, 1939; *National Ham and Eggs*, Oct. 14, Oct. 28, Nov. 4, 1939; Calif. [29], Oct. 1939, pp. 1, 5; Pasadena *Star-News*, Sept. 30, 1939; Santa Cruz *News*, Oct. 5, 1939. The Welfare Board's statement was based on the Social Security Act stipulations that aid granted under the act was to be paid in United States money and that the amount of aid given was to be based on need. Although the Ham and Eggs proposal satisfied neither stipulation, it was not intended to come under the Social Security Act or to replace it. This was pointed out in *National Ham and Eggs*, Sept. 30, Oct. 14, 1939. The board's statement, however, was probably very effective in helping to defeat the measure, since many recipients of old-age pensions were probably induced by fear of losing them to vote against Ham and Eggs.

103. Knepper, p. 58; Kenny, p. 132. For an effective attack on Ham and Eggs by a conservative Republican state senator, see John Phillips, *Inside California*, pp. 147–58.

104. Burke, p. 111.

105. For their efforts to gain support from other groups, see McWilliams, "Ham and Eggs," p. 332; *National Ham and Eggs*, June 10, July 1, Sept. 2, Oct. 7, Oct. 14, Oct. 28, Nov. 4, 1939. For mass meetings and entertainments of the time, see *ibid.*, July 8, Aug. 3, Sept. 9, Oct. 6, Nov. 5, 1939. Among the more flamboyant and seemingly profitable of the Ham and Eggs galas produced at this time were a bona fide traveling circus, a rodeo, and a Ham and Eggs revue entitled "Swing Your Ballot."

Ibid., July 29, Aug. 12, Aug. 26, Sept. 2, Sept. 9, Sept. 23, Oct. 7, Oct. 14, 1939.

106. *National Ham and Eggs*, Nov. 4, 1939; Knepper, p. 59. For the announcement about the warrants, see *National Ham and Eggs*, Sept. 30, 1939.

107. Calif. [53], Special Election, Nov. 7, 1939, p. 4.

108. San Francisco *Chronicle*, Oct. 27, 1939; *National Ham and Eggs*, Nov. 11, 1939.

109. *National Ham and Eggs*, Nov. 11, 1939.

110. *Ibid.*, Nov. 11, Nov. 18, 1939.

111. *Ibid.*, Nov. 18, Nov. 25, Dec. 2, 1939; Burke, p. 112.

112. *National Ham and Eggs*, Dec. 2, Dec. 23, 1939.

113. The Ham and Eggers joined forces with a recall movement already organized by a Los Angeles realtor, C. C. C. Tatum. *Ibid.*, Dec. 2, Dec. 9, Dec. 23, 1939, Jan. 27, 1940; Burke, pp. 149–50. The Ham and Eggs "candidate" to succeed Olson was Nathan T. Porter, who would later become a Townsend Party gubernatorial candidate. *National Ham and Eggs*, Nov. 18, 1939; O'Byrne, p. 149.

114. *National Ham and Eggs*, Dec. 9, Dec. 23, Dec. 30, 1939.

115. *Ibid.*, Feb. 3, 1940; San Francisco *Chronicle*, Jan. 30, Apr. 6, 1940.

116. Santa Cruz *News*, Nov. 13, 1939.

117. The other main defectors were Arthur C. Baer, C. J. Carpender, Roger Coffin, Fred Feighner, William Godsell, George Hankins, Eric Helgeson, Ray Howell, and Wayne Kintner. *National Ham and Eggs*, Jan. 6, Jan. 13, 1940; Los Angeles *Times*, Jan. 5, 1940. Apparently George McLain also left the organization at about this time, and in part because he opposed the recall movement, but his name was not mentioned in this connection by *National Ham and Eggs*. Pinner et al., pp. 33–34; McWilliams, "Pension Politics," p. 320.

118. *National Ham and Eggs*, Jan. 6, 1940.

119. Los Angeles *Times*, Jan. 5, 1940; *National Ham and Eggs*, Jan. 6, Jan. 13, Jan. 20, Mar. 23, Mar. 28, Apr. 4, Apr. 11, 1940; San Francisco *Chronicle*, Mar. 20, 1940; Santa Rosa *Press-Democrat*, Mar. 24, Apr. 26, May 8, May 9, 1940; Calif. [53], Presidential Primary, May 7, 1940; Burke, p. 149.

120. *National Ham and Eggs*, Feb. 24, Mar. 2, Apr. 11, Apr. 18, Apr. 25, May 16, May 23, June 27, 1940; Santa Rosa *Press-Democrat*, Mar. 17, Apr. 27, 1940.

121. Santa Rosa *Press-Democrat*, Jan. 6, 1940; Santa Cruz *News*, Nov. 20, 1939; *National Ham and Eggs*, Nov. 18, 1939; pamphlet of Initiative Defense League, 1940, in California State Library Collection of Campaign Literature.

122. *National Ham and Eggs*, July 4, July 11, July 18, July 25, Aug. 22, Aug. 29, 1940; *California Decisions*, Vol. 100, July–Nov. 1940, Decisions of week ending July 25, p. ii, Decisions of week ending Aug. 22, p. iii, Decisions of week ending Aug. 29, p. i.

123. The leadership endorsed congressional aspirants Tim Smith, Dis-

trict Eleven; Wolf Adler, District Thirteen; Samuel C. Converse, District Seventeen; and Harry E. Karst, District Sixteen. *National Ham and Eggs*, Aug. 22, 1940. For the vote count, see Calif. [53], Primary Election, Aug. 27, 1940, pp. 12, 14, 15.

124. *National Ham and Eggs*, Aug. 29, Sept. 12, Sept. 19, 1940.

125. For appeals for funds, see *ibid.*, Sept. 19, Oct. 17, 1940. For the declining number of meetings, see *ibid.*, June 27, July 25, Aug. 22, Sept. 26, Oct. 17, Nov. 7, 1940. The newspaper fell from twenty-four pages at the beginning of the year to twelve in May and eventually to four when the last issue was printed on June 6, 1941. On December 5, 1940, the paper's name was changed to *Economics Review*, and it retained this name until it expired.

126. *National Ham and Eggs*, Oct. 24, 1940.

CHAPTER 7

1. Calif. [9], pp. 712–14; Calif. [53], Primary Election, Aug. 30, 1938, p. 3.

2. Burke, pp. 3–4, 8–9.

3. *Ibid.*, p. 34.

4. Sacramento *Bee*, Jan. 2, 1939; Burke, p. 44.

5. Francis Carney, "The Rise of the Democratic Clubs in California," in Paul Tillett, ed., *Cases on Party Organization* (New York, 1963), pp. 34, 36.

6. Sacramento *Bee*, Jan. 2, 1939; Burke, p. 44.

7. Burke, pp. 64–65; Sacramento *Bee*, Jan. 3, Jan. 23, 1939.

8. Sacramento *Bee*, Jan. 10, 1939; Burke, pp. 59–60.

9. Burke, p. 68.

10. Quoted in *ibid.*, pp. 56–57. For the complete story of Olson and the Mooney affair, see *ibid.*, chap. 5, and Richard H. Frost, *The Mooney Case* (Stanford, Calif., 1968), chaps. 27, 28.

11. Burke, pp. 65–70; *Calaveras Prospect*, Apr. 15, 1939; Sacramento *Bee*, Jan. 2, Jan. 12, Jan. 16, Apr. 12, June 3, June 5, 1939.

12. For Olson's inaugural address see the Sacramento *Bee*, Jan. 3, 1939, and Burke, p. 12.

13. Sacramento *Bee*, Jan. 5, Jan. 12, Apr. 15, 1939; Santa Rosa *Press-Democrat*, Mar. 1, 1939. Some scholars agree with Olson that the aged have received a disproportionate amount of aid compared to other unfortunates since the Depression. See, for example, McHenry, p. 46, and Carlson, pp. 173–76.

14. At least two bills were introduced in this session to raise the maximum pension to $50 a month and lower the minimum age to 60. Several other radical proposals were made to raise pensions considerably more and to finance them by state lotteries, transactions taxes, or revenues gained from putting the state into the oil business. They were defeated on the grounds that they were too expensive and that California's old-age pension was already more generous than that of any other state. Sacramento *Bee*, Jan. 2, Jan. 3, Jan. 5, Jan. 14, Mar. 7, Mar. 8, Mar. 14, Apr. 7,

May 27, 1939; Burke, pp. 108–9; Peirce, pp. 87–88; U.S. [13], p. 25; Calif. [40], *AB*, 1939, ACA 51, AB 97; Calif. [42], *JA*, 53d sess., 1939, pp. 53, 70, 371, 2224, 2313, 2467, 2668, 2976, 2994, 3052, 3431–32, 3441–42. There was an actual increase in the maximum pension from $35 to $40 a month made effective January 1, 1940, but this came about mainly because of a 1939 amendment to the federal Social Security Act allowing federal reimbursements to states of up to one-half of a $40 pension. Calif. [24], July 1938–June 1940, p. 21; Holtzman, *Townsend Movement*, p. 105.

15. Sacramento *Bee*, June 15, June 21, 1939; Burke, p. 75. The Sonoma County Board, fearing that the county could not meet its age-old pension obligations unless it were given tax relief, specifically petitioned the Governor not to veto the bill. The same county's state senator, however, opposed the measure on the ground that the state could not afford to assume any more of the counties' obligations. Santa Rosa *Press-Democrat*, Jan. 25, Feb. 25, July 14, 1939.

16. Calif. [43], *JS*, 53d sess., 1939, pp. 329, 1000, 1018, 1213, 3132, 3157–58, 3192, 3193, 3214, 3226, 3401; Calif. [42], *JA*, 53d sess., 1939, pp. 1192, 1594, 2468, 2659, 2660–61, 3187, 3249; Calif. [46], *SB*, 1939, SB 780; Calif. [41], *Fin. Cal.*, 53d sess., 1939, p. 262. The bill was pocket-vetoed by the Governor.

17. *California Statutes*, 1939, chaps. 26, 52; Calif. [29], July 1939, p. 1; Sacramento *Bee*, Jan. 6, Jan. 24, Mar. 23, 1939. Governor Olson reputedly also appealed personally to President Roosevelt to sponsor the complete federal financing of old-age pensions. Pasadena *Star-News*, Dec. 16, 1938; San Francisco *Chronicle*, Dec. 18, 1938. Assemblyman Wilbur F. Gilbert of Los Angeles proposed a memorial asking Congress to lower the national pension age to 60, but this failed to pass. Calif. [42], *JA*, 53d sess., 1939, pp. 455, 3435; Calif. [40], *AB*, 1939, AJR 26.

18. Calif. [40], *AB*, 1939, AB 586; Calif. [42], *JA*, 53d sess., 1939, pp. 139, 479, 486–88, 512, 784, 795–98, 875, 1077, 1087–88, 1123, 1200, 1215–16, 1316, 1564, 1570–71, 1707, 1879, 2467–68, 2470, 3100, 3126, 3459; Calif. [43], *JS*, 53d sess., 1939, pp. 2450–51, 2670, 2736–37, 2821, 2872–73, 2956; Calif. [24], July 1938–June 1940, pp. 22–24; Calif. [29], Aug. 1939, p. 4.

19. This law was part of AB 586 in Calif. [40], *AB*, 1939. See also *California Statutes*, 1939, chap. 719. For the proposed constitutional amendment see Calif. [40], *AB*, 1939, ACA 1; Calif. [42], *JA*, 53d sess., 1939, pp. 70, 511, 812, 1813, 1969; Calif. [43], *JS*, 53d sess., 1939, pp. 877, 1620, 1717; and Calif. [29], July 1939, p. 1.

20. *California Welfare and Institutions Code*, sections 2226, 2229.

21. Calif. [24], July 1938–June 1940, pp. 22, 23.

22. *Ibid.*; Fitzgerald, p. 8.

23. "Many voters, infuriated by the defeat of Governor Olson's legislative program at the last session, are in no mood to debate the feasibility of the [Ham and Eggs] proposal. They are going to vote for the bill in blind despair, hoping against all reason that a miracle will occur and that the plan will work." McWilliams, "Ham and Eggs," p. 332.

24. Burke, p. 112; Santa Rosa *Press-Democrat*, Nov. 14, Nov. 15, 1939; Pasadena *Star News*, Nov. 16, 1939.

25. Santa Rosa *Press-Demócrat*, Nov. 16, Nov. 25, Nov. 26, 1939.

26. *Ibid.*, Nov. 22, Dec. 29, 1939; Santa Cruz *News*, Nov. 21, 1939; Pasadena *Star-News*, Dec. 28, 1939.

27. Santa Cruz *News*, Jan. 29, 1939. For Olson's program see also Burke, pp. 119–20; Santa Rosa *Press-Democrat*, Nov. 26, 1939; Long Beach *Press-Telegram*, Jan. 29, 1940; and Santa Cruz *News*, Jan. 24, 1939.

28. Sacramento *Bee*, Jan. 30, 1940; Burke, p. 121.

29. Burke, pp. 121–22; Long Beach *Press-Telegram*, Jan. 30, 1940; Santa Cruz *News*, Jan. 30, 1940.

30. Burke, pp. 126–38; Carlson, p. 169; Sacramento *Bee*, Feb. 3, Feb. 8, Feb. 12, Feb. 13, Feb. 21, Feb. 23, Feb. 24, Feb. 26, May 10, May 13, May 15, May 20–24, 1940.

31. The dictograph incident was revealed in the February 20, 1940, issue of the Sacramento *Bee*, and was investigated by a legislative committee. See Burke, pp. 123–26, and *Report of Assembly Investigating Committee on Interference with the Legislature, Including Minority Report and Reply to Minority Report Pursuant to House Resolutions Numbers 46 and 49* (Sacramento, 1940). For the defeat of Olson's legislative program see Burke, p. 123, and Sacramento *Bee*, Feb. 26, May 13, May 25, Sept. 19, 1940.

32. Sacramento *Bee*, Feb. 8, Feb. 15, Feb. 17, 1940; Calif. [40], *AB*, 1940, AB 95; Calif. [42], *JA*, 53d sess., 1940, pp. 164, 172, 278, 391–92, 971.

33. Sacramento *Bee*, Feb. 12, May 13, May 17, 1940. The legislature did pass another innocuous congressional memorial calling for a "uniform and liberal system of old-age assistance to be financed wholly from federal funds." Calif. [46], *SB*, 1940, SJR 1; Calif. [43], *JS*, 53d sess., 1st extra sess., 1940, pp. 57, 77–78, 124, 318, 328, 341; Calif. [42], *JA*, 53d sess., 1st extra sess., 1940, pp. 133, 249, 307, 357. The legislature refused, however, to pass a memorial endorsing the Townsend General Welfare Act, although Townsend himself addressed the legislature in its favor. Sacramento *Bee*, Feb. 20, 1940; *National Townsend Weekly*, June 1, 1940; Calif. [42], *JA*, 53d sess., 1st extra sess., 1940, pp. 577–78, 732–33, 891, 899, 971; Calif. [40], *AB*, 1940, AJR 24.

34. Calif. [29], May 1940, p. 6, July 1940, p. 5.

35. O'Byrne, p. 40.

36. San Francisco *Chronicle*, Oct. 15, 1939.

37. O'Byrne, p. 42; *National Townsend Weekly*, Dec. 1, 1939.

38. San Francisco *Chronicle*, Dec. 20, 1939.

39. *Ibid.*, Dec. 20, 1939, Jan. 5, 1940.

40. *Ibid.*, Dec. 20, 1939, Jan. 5, 1940, Jan. 20, 1939; Long Beach *Press-Telegram*, Jan. 25, 1940; *National Townsend Weekly*, Jan. 27, Feb. 3, 1940.

41. Santa Rosa *Press-Democrat*, Feb. 1, 1940; Calif. [46], *SB*, 1940, SB 57; Calif. [43], *JS*, 53d sess., 1st extra sess., 1940, pp. 87, 138, 142, 157–58, 170–71, 850.

42. Sacramento *Bee*, Feb. 7, Feb. 8, Feb. 12, Feb. 14, 1940; Calif. [42], *JA*, 53d sess., 1st extra sess., 1940, pp. 173, 234–35, 968.

43. Calif. [40], *AB*, 1940, AB 96; Calif. [42], *JA*, 53d sess., 1st extra sess., 1940, pp. 170, 172, 180–81, 312, 346, 975; Calif. [43], *JS*, 53d sess., 1st extra sess., 1940, pp. 178, 185, 234–35, 278–79; Sacramento *Bee*, Feb. 9, Feb. 10, Feb. 17, Feb. 19, 1940.

44. San Francisco *Chronicle*, Feb. 24, 1940; Sacramento *Bee*, Sept. 19, 1940.

45. Calif. [40], *AB*, 1940, ACA 6, AB 129; Calif. [42], *JA*, 53d sess., 1st extra sess., 1940, pp. 170, 173, 315, 374, 977; Calif. [43], *JS*, 53d sess., 1st extra sess., 1940, pp. 196, 202, 234, 235, 277; Sacramento *Bee*, Feb. 9, May 16, May 23, 1940.

46. Calif. [53], General Election, Nov. 5, 1940, p. 26.

47. See summary of California politics in the year 1940 by state senator Herbert W. Slater, Santa Rosa *Press-Democrat*, Dec. 31, 1940.

48. O'Byrne, pp. 43, 160–61; *National Townsend Weekly*, May 4, May 18, June 8, June 22, July 20, 1940.

49. *California Reports*, 2d ser., Vol. XVI (San Francisco, 1941), 276–85. California welfare officials were of the opinion that this decision rendered Proposition Two unnecessary. Calif. [29], Oct. 1940, p. 5, Nov. 1940, p. 1. They were probably in error, however, for the court decision merely upheld the right of county boards to release liens, whereas Proposition Two required them to do so. Proposition Two would thus be in line with the federal Social Security uniformity rule, whereas the court decision probably was not.

50. Calif. [53], General Election, Nov. 5, 1940, p. 26. There was doubt in some quarters about whether these constitutional amendments invalidated county liens taken before September 1, 1937, the date of the first lien repeal law. These doubts were stilled on November 22, 1940, when the Attorney General ruled that such liens were also invalidated by the passage of propositions One and Two. Calif. [29], Jan. 1940, p. 2, Nov. 1940, p. 1, Dec. 1940, p. 4.

51. This $38 pension was nearly twice the national average ($19.96), almost five times larger than the lowest pension ($8.01 in Georgia), and nearly $10 higher than the next highest pension ($28.59 in Massachusetts). Calif. [24], July 1938–June 1940, p. 25.

52. Calif. [5], p. 2004.

53. Bond et al., inside front cover.

54. AAOAS, *Thirteenth National Conference*, p. 170. California was outranked in per capita cost, however, by Colorado, with a per capita cost of $12.91. *Ibid.*; see also Bond et al., p. 68.

55. Bond et al., inside front cover and pp. 67–68; Calif. [24], July 1938–June 1940, pp. 19, 25, 27, and July 1940–June 1942, p. 15; U.S. [13], p. 24.

56. Warren won the support of several pension spokesmen, including the former Ham and Eggs leaders and George McLain. Burke, pp. 221–22, 223; see also Cresap, p. 102.

CHAPTER 8

1. California continues to pass much old-age legislation despite the fact that the proportion of old people in California has fallen below the national average since 1960 and will probably continue to fall in the future. U.S. [5], p. 6; Albrecht, "Sociological Impact of Aging," p. 1124.

2. For evidence of the continuing socioeconomic deprivation and political instability of the aged in California after 1940 see Pinner et al., chap. 3, and McWilliams, "Pension Politics," pp. 321–22. By "progressivism" I mean the active and widespread use of state governmental power to deal with public problems, especially problems of social welfare. According to one source, the social welfare program of Governor Brown's first administration was "the most progressive program of achievement in two decades." Calif. [33].

3. For a description of some of the new pension organizations that sprang up in the 1940's, see Calif. [44], Pt. I, pp. 61–66, and Pinner et al., pp. 4–5.

4. My account of McLain's life draws heavily on Pinner et al., pp. 23–46. See also "A Place in the Sun," p. 50.

5. Pinner et al., pp. 34–36; Calif. [44], pp. 60–61.

6. Pinner et al., pp. 39–46. The present organization is tied in with the National League of Senior Citizens, also founded by McLain. At one time the league had chapters in at least 29 states, but in recent years the number seems to have dwindled to about 10. *Senior Citizens Sentinel,* May 1964, Feb. 1970.

7. Pinner et al., pp. 243–50; Bond et al., pp. 81–87; Calif. [24], July 1948–June 1950, pp. 13–15.

8. Calif. [24], July 1948–June 1950, pp. 13–15; Pinner et al., chap. 6; Bond et al., pp. 87–91; California Constitution Revision Commission, *Article XXVII, Repeal of Article XXV, Old-Age Security and Security for the Blind, Background Study* (mimeo.; San Francisco, Mar. 1968).

9. Calif. [53], Presidential Primary Election, June 7, 1960, pp. 3–4. On March 6, 1964, McLain announced his candidacy for the United States Senate on a platform reminiscent of both the EPIC and Townsend movements. It proposed to "end poverty in America" by guaranteeing every aged person a minimum income of $216.50 a month, thereby "put[ting] every jobless American back to work to meet the new consumer demands of these elderly, hitherto neglected citizens." *Senior Citizens Sentinel,* May 1964. In this election, however, McLain was badly beaten.

10. New York *Times* (Western ed.), Sept. 9, 1963, p. 10; Totten J. Anderson and Eugene C. Lee, "The 1962 Election in California," *Western Political Quarterly,* XVI (1963), 409.

11. New York *Times* (Western ed.), Sept. 9, 1963; p. 10; *Senior Citizens Sentinel,* June, Sept. 1963; *Maturity,* Mar. 1962. One should not exaggerate the apparent closeness of Brown and McLain, however, for their relationship probably contained more elements of expediency than real warmth. An interview with Myrtle Williams on March 19, 1970, revealed

a greater attachment to Brown's predecessor, Goodwin Knight, on the part of the CLSC leadership, and a tendency to criticize Brown as an opportunist who gladly took credit for progressive old-age welfare legislation while doing little to secure its passage.

12. For a sophisticated analysis of McLain's entire organization and method of operation, see Pinner et al. Another useful account is Bond et al., pp. 78–104.

13. Pinner et al., pp. 250–56. McLain and his associates were busily lobbying in Sacramento at the time of his death and probably contributed importantly to the passage of some 45 enactments beneficial to the older age groups in the 1965 legislative session. *Senior Citizens Sentinel*, Jan., May, Aug. 1965; *Maturity*, Feb. 1966, supplement. Closely akin to lobbying activities on behalf of the aged is the McLain organization's "welfare service," which helps members apply for pensions and secure maximum grants and so on under the complex Old-Age Security Act. This service seems to be very effectively managed. Pinner et al., pp. 250–56.

14. Calif. [24], July 1940–June 1942, p. 15, and July 1950–June 1952, p. 31. This increase was not entirely steady over the ten-year period, for during 1942 and 1943 the number of aged welfare recipients declined, owing primarily to the improved economic conditions brought on by World War II. *Ibid.*, July 1940–June 1942, pp. 13–15, and July 1942–June 1944, p. 17.

15. *Ibid.*, July 1950–June 1952, p. 31; Calif. [21], 1964–65, Table 1, and 1965–66, Table 1; letter to the author from John M. McCoy, Chief, Program Estimates Bureau, Calif. Dept. of Social Welfare, Sept. 25, 1969.

16. Calif. [20], July 1957–June 1958, p. 5.

17. U.S. [16], p. 5; *Social Security Unemployment Compensation*, pp. 32505–32508.

18. Bond et al., inside front cover; Calif. [20], July 1954–June 1955, pp. 19–20, and July 1959–June 1960, pp. 13–14; Calif. [26], p. 8. The two categories of aged aid are not mutually exclusive, since many Californians draw both federal and state old-age pensions.

19. Calif. [24], July 1940–June 1942, p. 15, and July 1950–June 1952, p. 31; letter to the author from John M. McCoy, Chief, Program Estimates Bureau, Calif. Dept. of Social Welfare, Sept. 25, 1969.

20. Calif. [24], July 1940–June 1942, pp. 9–10, July 1942–June 1944, pp. 13–14, and July 1944–June 1946, p. 11.

21. *Ibid.*, July 1944–June 1946, p. 12, July 1946–June 1948, p. 10, and July 1948–June 1950, p. 13; Calif. [20], July 1954–June 1955, p. 18, and July 1956–June 1957, p. 13. The change from $65 to $75 in 1949 came as a result of the passage of McLain's radical initiative amendment in 1948. When the amendment was repealed by the voters the following year, the grant increase was specifically retained. Calif. [24], July 1948–June 1950, p. 13. For a thorough record of the Warren administration's backing of higher old-age pensions in the 1940's and early 1950's, see the newspaper clipping file in the Lyon Papers.

22. Calif. [20], July 1956–June 1957, p. 13.

23. *Ibid.*, July 1956–June 1957, p. 13, and July 1958–June 1959, pp. 15, 16; Calif. [26], p. 47; Calif. [38], p. 14; *Senior Citizens Sentinel*, Sept. 1963, Nov. 1969.

24. Calif. [24], July 1940–June 1942, p. 15, and July 1950–June 1952, p. 31; letter to the author from John M. McCoy, Chief, Program Estimates Bureau, Calif. Dept. of Social Welfare, Sept. 25, 1969.

25. Calif. [24], July 1942–June 1944, pp. 11, 15, July 1944–June 1946, pp. 12, 13, July 1946–June 1948, pp. 10, 12, July 1948–June 1950, p. 15, and July 1950–June 1952, p. 27; Calif. [20], July 1954–June 1955, pp. 18–19, and July 1957–June 1958, p. 5; Calif. [33], p. 7; *Maturity*, Sept. 1962, Aug. 1966; McLain; Calif. [8], p. 7. There were a few enactments during the 1950 and 1951 legislative sessions that tightened property and income restrictions, but they were of minor significance. Calif. [24], July 1950–June 1952, pp. 24, 25.

26. Calif. [24], July 1942–June 1944, p. 11, and July 1950–June 1952, p. 24; Calif. [20], July 1953–June 1954, p. 16; Calif. [26], p. 47; *Senior Citizens Sentinel*, Aug. and Apr. 1965, Mar. 1968. A state investigating committee noted that the virtual elimination of the clause was essential in "alleviating undue hardships upon sons and daughters and removing strain on family ties of aged persons." Calif. [38], p. 14.

27. Calif. [38], p. 14; Calif. [20], July 1954–June 1955, p. 18.

28. Calif. [24], July 1940–June 1942, p. 11, July 1942–June 1944, pp. 12, 13, July 1944–June 1946, p. 12, July 1946–June 1948, p. 10, and July 1950–June 1952, p. 25; Calif. [20], July 1953–June 1954, pp. 12–13, 16, July 1958–June 1959, pp. 13–16, and July 1959–June 1960, pp. 14–15; *Maturity*, Dec. 1962 and July 1963; McLain. The most important recent breakthrough in this respect has been the adoption of the "declaration of need" system for OAS applicants, which enables them to begin drawing pensions immediately on applying without waiting for cumbersome investigations of their finances to be completed. Instead, a spot-check system similar to that of the Bureau of Internal Revenue is used. *Senior Citizens Sentinel*, Dec. 1966; *Los Angeles Times*, Nov. 21, 1968; Calif. Dept. of Social Welfare, *Department Bulletin*, no. 651.

29. Calif. [24], July 1948–June 1950, pp. 15–16.

30. Calif. [20], July 1956–June 1957, p. 14.

31. Calif. [39].

32. *Maturity*, May 1962. The practice of designating May as Senior Citizens Month was repeated by Brown in subsequent years and has been continued by Reagan. *Maturity*, May 1964, Aug. 1966; *Senior Californian*, Vol. I, nos. 1, 5.

33. *Maturity*, May 1962.

34. *Ibid.*, Sept. 1962.

35. Calif. [24], July 1948–June 1950, p. 16, and July 1950–June 1952, p. 27.

36. *Ibid.*, July 1950–June 1952, pp. 27–28; Calif. [23].

37. Calif. [20], July 1958–June 1959, p. 15, and July 1959–June 1960,

pp. 15–16. The official purpose of SB 437 was to use community organizations and resources to give older persons "an opportunity to remain active and contributing members in their community to the fullest extent possible." Calif. [27], p. 1. The projects envisioned by the act were providing skilled social workers and other trained persons to serve the aged; developing employment opportunities; establishing "senior citizen centers" of all kinds; enabling aged persons to remain in their home communities or to return there from institutions; establishing home-finding and placement services; financing leadership courses for aged persons; expanding library services for the aged; acquainting communities with the problems of aging; conducting surveys on community needs and resources in aiding the aged; and many others. *Ibid.*, pp. 1–2.

38. Calif. [38], p. 15; *Maturity*, May, Sept. 1962, July, Nov. 1964; Calif. [8], pp. 4–6, 13–14; Calif. [6].

39. Calif. [6], p. 11; Calif. [8], p. 9; Calif. [38], pp. 8–9; U.S. [16], p. 23; Sacramento *Bee*, Aug. 5, 1959; Sacramento *Union*, Aug. 10, 1959. The state had made some effort to work out an effective employment program for the aged during World War II and the Korean War, but its efforts were not very successful. Calif. [24], July 1942–June 1944, pp. 12–13, July 1944–June 1946, p. 14, and July 1950–June 1952, pp. 26–27.

40. Calif. [38], pp. 7–8; Calif. [6], p. 14. For an illuminating exchange on the pros and cons of the adult education program for the aged, see letters to the editor by Henry C. MacArthur and Louis Kuplan in the Palo Alto *Times*, Mar. 23, Apr. 2, 1959.

41. In November 1968 the Los Angeles County Board of Supervisors, usually a conservative body, passed a resolution to that effect. *Senior Citizens Sentinel*, Nov. 1968. The recent United States Supreme Court decision invalidating state residence requirements for welfare applicants has probably further strengthened sentiment for this solution.

42. This proposal was originally introduced in Congress by California Representative James Roosevelt in 1963 to guarantee a minimum income of $199 a month to its beneficiaries. Its present sponsor is California Congressman Phillip Burton, whose bill would raise benefits to $277 a month. It has many avowed proponents in California, including the Los Angeles County Board of Supervisors and United States Senator Alan Cranston. *Senior Citizens Sentinel*, Jan. 1964, Nov., Dec. 1968, Feb., Mar., May, July, Aug., Oct. 1969. A recent survey shows that most OAS caseworkers in California are also in favor of it. Calif. [35], p. 14.

43. *Senior Citizens Sentinel*, May, July 1965, Feb., Oct. 1969; Calif. [6], p. 16.

44. *Senior Citizens Sentinel*, Oct., Nov. 1965, Feb., May 1969; Calif. [32], Statistical Series PA3-117, June 1969, tables 12–14a.

45. *Maturity*, May 1965, Feb. 1966.

46. *Ibid.*, Feb. 1966; *Senior Citizens Sentinel*, July 1969.

47. Calif. [24], July 1940–June 1942, pp. 11–12, and July 1944–June 1946, pp. 12–13.

48. Calif. [20], July 1954–June 1955, p. 19.

49. In October 1955 the state began to subsidize pensioners' medical

care in county hospitals for as long as they needed it, and to make direct payments to "vendors" of medical services who ministered to pensioners' needs. *Ibid.*, July 1955–June 1956, p. 25, and July 1959–June 1960, p. 14.

50. *Ibid.*, July 1957–June 1958, p. 6; Calif. [26], pp. 16–17; Calif. [48], p. 13. The program applied to beneficiaries of the state's Aid to the Blind, Aid to the Needy Children, and Aid to the Needy Disabled programs as well as to OAS recipients. The pensioners, however, made the heaviest demands on it.

51. Calif. [26], pp. 17–18; Calif. [48], pp. 13–14. California participated enthusiastically in the program and received a major share of the federal funds. Greenfield, *Medicare and Medicaid*, pp. 69–70.

52. Calif. [6], pp. 15–17.

53. *Ibid.*; Calif. [18], pp. 6–7.

54. *Medicare and Social Security Explained*, pp. 141, 161, and *passim*; *Social Security Unemployment Compensation*, pp. 32507–32508; Greenfield, *Medicare and Medicaid*.

55. U.S. [19], pp. 20–23, tables 22–25; Greenfield, *Medicare and Medicaid*, pp. 28–30. On shortcomings in the act see *ibid.*, pp. 42–50.

56. Greenfield, *Medicare and Medicaid*, p. v and chaps. 4–5.

57. *Maturity*, Aug. 1966; Calif. [8], p. 13; Calif. [16], p. 7. The liberal provisions for psychiatric treatment for the aged may, however, intensify the already serious trend of committing aged persons to mental hospitals unnecessarily. Recent legislation has been passed to curb this trend. Calif. [6], p. 12; *Maturity*, Feb. 1965; *Senior Citizens Sentinel*, Aug., Oct. 1967.

58. Calif. [50], nos. 68-7, 68-8, 68-9, 69-1.

59. Letter to the author from John M. McCoy, Chief, Program Estimates Bureau, Calif. Dept. of Social Welfare, Sept. 25, 1969. Again it should be remembered that in both cases about half the total outlay came from the federal government.

60. Greenfield, *Medicare and Medicaid*, pp. 127–28.

61. Calif. [47], pp. 15–19; Calif. [50], no. 68-1; Calif. [49], nos. 6, 7.

62. In November 1966 some 34 per cent of the population of the CLSC Senior Citizens Village in Fresno voted for Reagan. A year later a CLSC poll indicated that 95 per cent of the organization's membership rated Reagan's performance as "poor," and by March 1968 the same percentage wanted him recalled. *Senior Citizens Sentinel*, Nov. 1967, Mar., Nov. 1968.

63. *Ibid.*, Mar. 1967, Jan. 1968.

64. *Ibid.*, Oct., Dec. 1967.

65. *Ibid.*, Nov. 1966.

66. On employment see *Senior Californian*, Vol. I, no. 2 (1968), and Los Angeles *Times*, June 10, Oct. 29, 1969. On tax relief see *Senior Citizens Sentinel*, Sept. 1967; Calif. [37]; *Senior Californian*, Vol. I, nos. 1, 2; and Calif. [45].

67. Greenfield, *Medicare and Medicaid*, pp. 45–46; *Senior Citizens Sentinel*, Dec. 1965; *Newsletter of the Friends Committee on Legislation*, XVIII, 8 (Aug.-Sept. 1969), 5.

68. *Senior Citizens Sentinel*, Dec. 1966.

69. *Ibid.*, Mar. 1967.

70. *Ibid.*, June, July, Aug., Sept., Oct. 1967.

71. *Ibid.*, Jan., Feb., Mar., July, Aug., Sept., Oct. 1968; Los Angeles *Times*, July 28, Sept. 19, 1968.

72. *Senior Citizens Sentinel*, July, Aug. 1967; Los Angeles *Times*, Oct. 31, 1969.

73. A detailed exposition of the Governor's views on this subject, in which he was supported in part by some members of the legislature, can be found in Calif. [11], pp. 4–7, 10, and in Calif. [47], pp. 8, 10, 20–21.

74. *Senior Citizens Sentinel*, Mar., June, Dec. 1967.

75. *Ibid.*, Sept., Oct. 1967, Jan., Feb. 1968; Los Angeles *Times*, Feb. 7, Feb. 22, May 3, Aug. 1, 1968, Nov. 4, 1969, Mar. 20, 1970; Budget Message from the Governor of California, Feb. 4, 1969, p. vii.

76. *Senior Citizens Sentinel*, Mar. 1968, Feb., Apr., May, June, July 1969; Los Angeles *Times*, July 3, 1968, May 6, 1969.

77. *Senior Citizens Sentinel*, Sept. 1969.

78. *Ibid.*, Nov. 1969, Feb. 1970; Santa Ana *Register*, Oct. 17, 1969.

79. When a federal court outlawed the residence requirement for welfare recipients, some Reagan administration officials reportedly charged that this decision would bring an army of indigents, aged and otherwise, into the state to enjoy California's "generous" welfare and OAS benefits. *Senior Citizens Sentinel*, June 1968; Los Angeles *Times*, May 11, 1968. On March 19, 1970, Reagan proposed that the state limit the amount of welfare payment, including OAS grants, made to a new resident to the amount he would have received in his home state, until he had lived in California for a full year. Los Angeles *Times*, Mar. 20, 1970.

80. *Maturity*, Mar. 1963, May 1965; U.S. [19]; Burger, p. 14; Calif. [4], pp. 7–10; Los Angeles *Times*, Sept. 28, 1969.

81. Calif. [28], pp. 2–3; Burger, p. 14; Calif. [17], pp. 117–25; Los Angeles *Times*, Oct. 24, 1969. For a less gloomy view of the health problems of America's aged, see Rosow, pp. 3–4.

82. On substandard nursing homes in California and for instances of aged patients' being exploited under Medi-Cal, see *Senior Citizens Sentinel*, July 1965; Los Angeles *Times*, Sept. 30, 1969; Calif. [45]; and Burger, pp. 16–17. For a withering but largely undocumented attack on the nursing-home "racket" in the United States, see Garvin and Burger. For a more favorable view, see California Association of Homes for the Aging, *Trends and Topics*, and Calif. [25], pp. 1–11.

83. *Maturity*, Dec. 1962, Feb. 1964; U.S. [16], pp. 24–25; Calif., Governor's Advisory Commission on Housing Problems: *Report on Housing in California* (Sacramento, 1963), pp. 36–38; *Summary of Housing in California* (Sacramento, 1963), p. 5; *Appendix to the Report on Housing in California* (Sacramento, 1963), pp. 617–48.

84. Burger.

85. Garvin and Burger, p. 142.

86. *Ibid.*, p. 149.

87. U.S. [19], p. 4.

88. Rosow, p. 5.

89. *Ibid.* Rosow's entire book is a sophisticated and persuasive elaboration of this thesis. See also Calif. [25], pp. 2, 10, and California Association of Homes for the Aging, *Trends and Topics*, no. 3, pp. 3–19. Lakeport in northern California is an example of a "natural" retirement community that is apparently entirely satisfactory to the aged. Los Angeles *Times*, Sept. 3, 1968.

90. *Senior Citizens Sentinel*, Oct. 1969. McLain attempted to establish a second Senior Citizens Village in Antelope Valley, Calif., in 1963, but the effort failed for lack of funds. *Ibid.*, Sept., Oct., Dec. 1963, Feb. 1964; New York *Times* (Western ed.), Sept. 9, 1963; Garvin and Burger, p. 140. The CLSC also agitates for increases in rental allowances under OAS and for the abolition of home-occupancy deductions from OAS checks. *Senior Citizens Sentinel*, Jan. 1969.

91. The quotation is from Dr. Vern Bengston, Univ. of Southern Calif. Gerontology Center, quoted in *Senior Californian*, Vol. I, no. 3, p. 4. For a similar presentation from the same center, see Los Angeles *Times*, Aug. 18, 1968.

92. For evidence of a greater awareness of, and sympathy for, the problems of the aged in California, see Donahue and Tibbitts, pp. 51–53.

93. *Senior Californian*, Vol. I, no. 5. For a blistering attack on this proclamation as being hypocritical, see *Senior Citizens Sentinel*, Oct. 1969.

94. Los Angeles *Times*, Jan. 12, Mar. 31, 1969. The CLSC argues that, on the contrary, federal poverty programs do not provide for old people at all. *Senior Citizens Sentinel*, Apr. 1966.

95. On proposals to reinstate the property lien and relative-responsibility provisions, see *Senior Citizens Sentinel*, Mar., Sept. 1964, Mar., June 1965, May 1966; and Calif. [48], pp. 48–50. On opposition to efforts to simplify OAS procedures, see *Senior Citizens Sentinel*, Oct. 1965, Apr., June 1966, Apr. 1967, Feb. 1968, Mar. 1969; Los Angeles *Times*, Jan. 29, Mar. 12, Mar. 27, 1968, Feb. 28, 1969. On lie-detector tests, see *Senior Citizens Sentinel*, Dec. 1964, and for the quotation, see *ibid.*, Mar. 1965.

Bibliography

Bibliography

In this Bibliography California and United States government publications are identified by bracketed numbers for convenience in citation.

"Agitation for Pension and Scrip Schemes," *Editorial Research Reports,* II (1938), 227–44.

Albrecht, Ruth. "The Social Roles of Old People," *Journal of Gerontology,* VI (1951), 138–45.

———. "The Sociological Impact of Aging on Present-Day Culture," *Physical Therapy,* XLVIII (1968), 1123–28.

Alsop, Joseph, and Robert Kintner. "Merchandising Miracles: Sheridan Downey and the Pension Business," *Saturday Evening Post,* Sept. 16, 1939, pp. 5–7, 85–87, 89–90.

Altmeyer, Arthur J. The Formative Years of Social Security. 2d printing. Madison: Univ. of Wis. Press, 1968.

American Association for Old-Age Security (AAOAS). Old-Age Security Progress: Report of the Proceedings of the Fourth National Conference on Old-Age Security. New York: AAOAS, 1931.

———. Old-Age Security in the United States, 1932: A Record of the Fifth National Conference on Old-Age Security. New York: AAOAS, 1932.

———. Social Security in the United States: A Record of the Sixth National Conference on Old-Age and Social Security. New York: AAOAS, 1933.

———. Social Security in the United States, 1934: A Record of the Seventh National Conference on Social Security. New York: AAOAS, 1934.

———. Social Security in the United States, 1940: A Record of the Thirteenth National Conference on Social Security. New York: AAOAS, 1940.

Andrews, Irene Osgood. "Pensions for the Oldest," *American Labor Legislation Review,* XIX (1929), 294–95.

Bakersfield *Californian.* For the years 1920–40.

Bancroft, Philip. "Politics, Farming, and the Progressive Party in California." Univ. of Calif., Berkeley, Regional Cultural History Project, 1962.

Typescript. A copy is also to be found in the Univ. of Calif., Los Angeles, Library, Dept. of Special Collections.

Bancroft Library Collection of Campaign Literature from the California Elections of 1934 and 1938. Univ. of Calif., Berkeley.

Barron, Milton L. "Minority Group Characteristics of the Aged in American Society," *Journal of Gerontology*, VIII (1953), 477–82.

Barton, Bruce. "How to Fix Everything," *Vanity Fair*, Aug. 1931, pp. 31, 70.

Beman, Lamar T., ed. Selected Articles on Old-Age Pensions. New York: H. W. Wilson, 1927.

Bennett, David H. Demagogues in the Depression: American Radicals and the Union Party, 1932–1936. New Brunswick, N.J.: Rutgers Univ. Press, 1969.

Berelson, Bernard P., et al. Voting: A Study of Opinion Formation in a Presidential Campaign. Chicago: Univ. of Chicago Press, 1954.

Berwick, Keith. "The 'Senior Citizen' in America: A Study in Unplanned Obsolescence," *The Gerontologist*, VII (1967), 257–60.

Birren, James E., and Vern L. Bengston. "The Young, the Old, and the In-Between," *Center Magazine*, Mar. 1969, pp. 84–86.

Blackorby, Edward C. Prairie Rebel: The Public Life of William Lemke. Lincoln: Univ. of Nebr. Press, 1963.

Blau, Zena Smith. "Old Age: A Study of Change in Status." Ph.D. diss., Columbia Univ., 1957.

Bond, Floyd A., et al. Our Needy Aged: A California Study of A National Problem. New York: Holt, 1954.

Boone, Andrew R. "Who Is Roy Owens?" *California, Magazine of the Pacific*, Sept. 1938, pp. 13, 30–31.

Bornet, Vaughn D. California Social Welfare: Legislation, Financing, Services, Statistics. Englewood Cliffs, N.J.: Prentice-Hall, 1956.

———. Welfare in America. Norman: Univ. of Okla. Press, 1960.

Bromley, Dennis B. The Psychology of Human Ageing. Baltimore: Penguin, 1966.

Burger, Robert E. "Who Cares for the Aged?" *Saturday Review*, Jan. 29, 1969, pp. 14–17.

Burke, Robert E. Olson's New Deal for California. Berkeley: Univ. of Calif. Press, 1953.

Cahn, Francis, and Valeska Bary. Welfare Activities of Federal, State, and Local Governments in California, 1850–1934. Berkeley: Univ. of Calif. Press, 1936.

Cain, James M. "Paradise," *American Mercury*, XXVIII (1933), 266–80.

Calaveras Prospect (San Andreas, Calif.). For the years 1920–40.

California, State of, government publications. Published in Sacramento unless otherwise noted.

[1] Board of Charities and Corrections. Biennial Report. For the years 1918–22.

[2] Citizens Advisory Committee on Aging. California's Older Population: Projections, 1960–1968. 1963.

[3] ———. *Maturity.* Newsletter of Citizens Advisory Committee on Aging. For the years 1953–67. Cited in the Notes as *Maturity.*

[4] ———. Report to the California Legislature on Age Discrimination in Public Agencies. 1966.

[5] Citizens State-Wide Committee on Old-Age Pensions. Report. California Legislature, Journal of the Assembly, 55th sess., 1943, Vol. I, pp. 1953–2059.

[6] Commission on Aging. Directory of Senior Centers and Special Services for Older Californians. 1966.

[7] ———. *Senior Californian.* For the years 1968–69. Cited in the Notes as *Senior Californian.*

[8] ———. Ten Years of Progress for Older Californians, 1956–1966. 1966.

[9] Department of Finance. California Blue Book. 1958.

[10] ———. Program Support and Local Assistance Budget for the Fiscal Year July 1, 1969, to June 30, 1970. 1969.

[11] ———. "State of California Fiscal Outlook for 1968–1969." Dec. 11, 1967. Mimeo.

[12] ———. Support and Local Assistance Budget for the Fiscal Year July 1, 1967, to June 30, 1968. 1967.

[13] ———. Support and Local Assistance Budget for the Fiscal Year July 1, 1968, to June 30, 1969. 1968.

[14] Department of Industrial Relations. Middle Aged and Older Workers. Special Bulletin no. 1. San Francisco, Jan. 1930.

[15] ———. Middle Aged and Older Workers in California. Special Bulletin no. 2. San Francisco, Aug. 1930.

[16] Department of Mental Hygiene. Medicare, Medi-Cal, and the Psychiatric Patient. Jan. 1967.

[17] ———. Mental Health Problems of Public Assistance Clients, A Mental Health Planning Study. June 1967.

[18] Department of Public Health. California's Older People — Their Health Problems. 1965.

[19] Department of Public Welfare. Biennial Report, July 1, 1924–June 30, 1926, With Additional Data, 1922–1924. 1927.

[20] Department of Social Welfare. Annual Report. For the years 1953–62.

[21] ———. Annual Statistical Report. For the years 1963–68.

[22] ———. Background Material for the Governor's Conference on Aging. 1960.

[23] ———. Background Material for the Governor's Conference on the Problems of the Aging. 1951.

[24] ———. Biennial Report. For the years 1927–52.

[25] ———. California Homes for the Aging. Report Requested by House Resolution No. 517—1967 Legislature. 1968.

[26] ———. "California's Public Welfare Programs and Problems." Oct. 1961. Mimeo.

[27] ———. "Community Service Projects for Older Persons." 1961. Mimeo.

[28] ———. An Expanded Program of Medical Care for the Poor: Program Planning Report no. 1. Aug. 1965.

[29] ———. *News Bulletin.* May 1932–Dec. 1940.

[30] ———. Old-Age Dependency: A Study of the Care Given to the Needy Aged in California. 1928.

[31] ———. Public Assistance in California, Jan. 1937–Dec. 1940.

[32] ———. Public Welfare in California. Statistical Series PA3–96, Sept. 1967; PA3–117, June 1969.

[33] ———. "Record of Achievements, January 1959–July 1961." N.d. Mimeo.

[34] ———. Significant Facts about Old-Age Security Recipients. Feb. 1957.

[35] ———. A Survey of California's Old-Age Security Caseworkers. June 1969.

[36] ———. What's New for California's Senior Citizens? 1961.

[37] Franchise Tax Board. A Summary of the California Senior Citizens Property Tax Assistance Law, 1968. 1968.

[38] Interdepartmental Committee on Problems of the Aging. "Annual Report to Governor Edmund G. Brown." 1962. Mimeo.

[39] ———. California Cares about Its Elder Citizens. 1962.

[40] Legislature. Assembly Bills.

[41] ———. Final Calendar of Legislative Business. For the years 1921–68.

[42] ———. *Journal of the Assembly.* For the years 1921–68.

[43] ———. *Journal of the Senate.* For the years 1921–68.

[44] ———. Report of the Senate Interim Committee on Social Welfare. 1949.

[45] ———. Report to the People. 1969.

[46] ———. Senate Bills.

[47] ———, Assembly Committee on Public Health. A Preliminary Report on Medi-Cal. Feb. 1968.

[48] ———, Senate Fact-Finding Committee on Labor and Welfare. California's Public Assistance Programs. 1965.

[49] Office of Health Care Services. Medical Care and Utilization Project Report. Nos. 5, 6, 7. N.d.

[50] ———. Medi-Cal Report. Nos. 68–1 (Apr. 10, 1968); 68–7, 68–8, 68–9 (all Dec. 1, 1968); 69–1 (Apr. 1969).

[51] ———. Public Welfare Medical Care in California from 1957 to 1966. 1966.

[52] Secretary of State. California Amendments to the Constitution and Proposed Statutes. For the years 1932–48.

[53] ———. Statement of Vote. For the years 1920–68.

California Association of Homes for the Aging. Trends and Topics: Guides to Policy and Action. Pamphlets no. 1, 2, 3. Sacramento, n.d.

"The California Old-Age Pension Law," *American Labor Legislation Review*, XIX (1929), 297.

"California Rescuing Her Aged," *American Labor Legislation Review*, XIX (1929), 68–73.

"California's Aged," *Survey*, LXI (1929), 781–82.

California State Chamber of Commerce. A Study of Facts Regarding Old-Age Aid Legislation and Costs. N.p., 1937.

California State Library Collection of Campaign Literature, Sacramento.

"California Triumphant," *Eagles Magazine*, XVII (July 1929), 5–7, 39–40.

Campbell, Angus, et al. The American Voter. New York: Wiley, 1960.

Canterbury, John H. " 'Ham and Eggs' in California," *The Nation*, CXLVII (1938), 408–10.

Cantril, Hadley. The Psychology of Social Movements. New York: Wiley, 1941.

Carlson, Oliver. A Mirror for Californians. Indianapolis, Ind.: Bobbs-Merrill, 1941.

Carp, Frances M. "Attitudes of Old Persons Toward Themselves and Toward Others," *Journal of Gerontology*, XXII (1967), 308–12.

Caughey, John W. California. Englewood Cliffs, N.J.: Prentice-Hall, 1953.

Cavan, Ruth S., et al. Personal Adjustment in Old Age. Chicago: Social Science Research Associates, 1949.

Chinn, Ronald E. "The Sinclair Campaign of 1934." M.A. thesis, Stanford Univ., 1937.

Clague, Ewan. "The Aging Population and Problems of Security," *Milbank Memorial Fund Quarterly*, XVIII (1940), 345–48.

Clark, John Gee. "John Gee Clark: California Legislator, Executive Administrator and Judge." Univ. of Calif., Los Angeles, Oral History Program, 1966. Typescript.

Cleland, Robert G. California in Our Time. New York: Knopf, 1947.

Conyngton, Mary. "Extent and Distribution of Old-Age Dependency in the United States," *Monthly Labor Review*, XXXVIII (1934), 1–10.

Corson, John J., and John W. McConnell. Economic Needs of Older People. Baltimore: Lord Baltimore Press, 1956.

Cowdry, E. V., ed. Problems of Ageing: Biological and Medical Aspects. Baltimore: Williams and Wilkins, 1939. 2d ed., 1942.

Creel, George. Rebel at Large: Recollections of Fifty Crowded Years. New York: Putnam, 1947.

———. "Utopia Unlimited," *Saturday Evening Post*, Nov. 24, 1934, pp. 5–7, 78–80.

Cresap, Dean R. Party Politics in the Golden State. Los Angeles: Haynes Foundation, 1954.

Crittenden, John. "Aging and Party Affiliation," *Public Opinion Quarterly*, XXVI (1962), 648–57.

———. "Aging and Political Participation," *Western Political Quarterly*, XVI (1963), 323–31.

Crouch, Winston W., et al. California Government and Politics. Englewood Cliffs, N.J.: Prentice-Hall, 1956.

Cumming, M. Elaine, and William E. Henry. Growing Old: The Process of Disengagement. New York: Basic Books, 1961.

Curtis, Howard J. "A Composite Theory of Aging," *The Gerontologist*, VI (1966), 143–49.

Daily Palo Alto Times. For the years 1920–60.

Derber, Milton, ed. The Aged and Society. Champaign, Ill.: Industrial Relations Research Association, 1950.

De Turbeville, Esther. "California Adopts Old-Age Pensions," *American Labor Legislation Review*, XIX (1929), 291–93.

Dodd, Paul A., and E. F. Penrose. Economic Aspects of Medical Services with Special Reference to Conditions in California. Washington, D.C.: Graphic Arts, 1939.

Donahue, Wilma, and Clark Tibbitts, eds. Politics of Age: Proceedings of the University of Michigan 14th Annual Conference on Aging, 1961. Ann Arbor: Univ. of Mich., 1962.

Dorman, Morgan J. Age before Booty: An Explanation of the Townsend Plan. New York: Putnam, 1936.

Downey, Sheridan. Highways to Prosperity. Chicago: Townsend National Weekly, 1940.

———. Onward America. Sacramento: Sheridan Downey, 1933.

———. Pensions or Penury? New York: Harper, 1939.

———. Why I Believe in the Townsend Plan. Sacramento: Sheridan Downey, 1936.

Drake, Joseph T. The Aged in American Society. New York: Ronald, 1958.

EPIC News (Los Angeles). For the years 1937–40. [Varying titles.]

Epstein, Abraham. The Challenge of the Aged. New York: Vanguard, 1928.

———. Facing Old Age: A Study of Old-Age Dependency in the United States and Old-Age Pensions. New York: Knopf, 1922.

———. Insecurity, A Challenge to America: A Study of Social Insurance in the United States and Abroad. New York: Harrison Smith and Robert Haas, 1933.

———. "Old-Age Pensions," *American Labor Legislation Review*, XII (1922), 221–27.

———. Old-Age Security. New York: League for Industrial Democracy, 1930.

———. "Present Status of Old-Age Pension Legislation in the United States," *Monthly Labor Review*, XIX (1924), 760–67.

———. "A Sidelight on the Family Status of Aged Dependents," *American Labor Legislation Review*, XV (1925), 30–31.

"Experience under State Old-Age Pension Laws in 1932," *Monthly Labor Review*, XXXVII (1933), 251–62.

"Extent of Old-Age Dependency," *Monthly Labor Review*, XXVI (1928), 960–62.

Fisher, Irving. "The Stamped Scrip Plan," *New Republic*, Dec. 21, 1932, pp. 163–64.

———. Stamp Scrip. New York: Adelphi, 1933.

Fitzgerald, Bill Edward. "Pension Politics in California." M.A. thesis, Univ. of Calif., Berkeley, 1951.

Ford, John Anson. Thirty Explosive Years in Los Angeles County. San Marino, Calif.: Huntington Library, 1961.

Frankhouser, William C. A Financial History of California: Public Revenues, Debts, and Expenditures. Berkeley: Univ. of Calif., 1913.

Fraternal Order of Eagles (FOE). Historic Words and Pens. South Bend, Ind.: FOE, 1934.

———. Social Security, the Eagles and the Social Security Act. N.p., n.d.

———, National Old-Age Pension Commission. Answers to Objections Advanced Against Old-Age Pensions. Milwaukee, Wis.: FOE, 1924.

Friedman, Eugene, and Robert J. Havighurst. The Meaning of Work and Retirement. Chicago: Univ. of Chicago Press, 1954.

Garvin, Richard, and Robert E. Burger. Where They Go to Die: The Tragedy of America's Aged. New York: Delacorte, 1968.

Gergen, Kenneth, and Kurt W. Back. "Aging, Time Perspective, and Preferred Solutions to International Conflicts," *Journal of Conflict Resolution*, IX (1965), 177–86.

"Gerontion," *Geriatrics,* V (1950), 338.

Gilbert, Jeanne G. Understanding Old Age. New York: Ronald, 1952.

Glane, Sam. "The Administration of Public Aid to Indigent Aged in California with Special Reference to Los Angeles County." M.S. thesis, Univ. of Southern Calif., 1937.

Glenn, Norval D. "Aging, Disengagement, and Opinionation," *Public Opinion Quarterly*, XXXIII (1969), 17–33.

Goldstein, Sidney. "Changing Income and Consumption Patterns of the Aged, 1950–1960," *Journal of Gerontology*, XX (1965), 453–61.

Grant, Margaret. Old-Age Security: Social and Financial Trends. Washington, D.C.: Social Science Research Council, 1939.

Greenfield, Margaret. Administration of Old-Age Security in California. Berkeley: Inst. of Governmental Studies, Univ. of Calif., 1950.

———. Medicare and Medicaid: The 1965 and 1967 Social Security Amendments. Berkeley: Inst. of Governmental Studies, Univ. of Calif., 1968.

Gusfield, Joseph R. "The Problem of Generations in Organizational Structure," *Social Forces*, XXXV (1957), 323–30.

Hall, G. Stanley. Senescence: The Last Half of Life. New York: Appleton, 1923.

Hamilton, Phil. "$30 a Week for Life!" *California, Magazine of the Pacific*, Aug. 1938, pp. 12–13, 36.

Hansen, Robert W. The Eagles. N.p., n.d.

————. Eagles Are People Helping People. FOE Personal Growth Leaflet no. 241. N.p., n.d.

Harris, Herbert. "Dr. Townsend's Marching Soldiers," *Current History*, XLIII (1936), 455–62.

Havighurst, Robert J. "Social and Psychological Needs of the Aging," *Annals of the American Academy*, CCLXXIX (1952), 11–17.

————. "A Social-Psychological Perspective on Aging," *The Gerontologist*, VIII (1968), 67–71.

————, and Ruth Albrecht. Older People. New York: Longmans, Green, 1953.

Heller Committee for Research in Social Economics of the University of California. The Dependent Aged in San Francisco. Berkeley: Univ. of Calif., 1928.

Hitt, Homer L. "The Role of Migration in Population Change among the Aged," *American Sociological Review*, XIX (1954), 194–200.

Holtzman, Abraham. "Analysis of Old-Age Politics in the United States," *Journal of Gerontology*, IX (1954), 56–66.

————. The Townsend Movement: A Political Study. New York: Bookman, 1963.

————. "The Townsend Movement: A Study in Old-Age Pressure Politics." Ph.D. diss. Harvard Univ., 1952.

"Hot Money for Californians," *California, Magazine of the Pacific*, Sept. 1938, pp. 12, 26–29.

Hyink, Bernard, Seyom Brown, and Ernest W. Thacker. Politics and Government in California. New York, Crowell, 1961.

Imperial Valley Press (El Centro, Calif.). For the years 1920–40.

Jacobs, Clyde, and John F. Gallagher. California Government: One among Fifty. New York: Macmillan, 1966.

Jones, Herbert C. "On California Government and Public Issues." Univ. of Calif., Berkeley, Regional Cultural History Project, 1957.

Kastenbaum, Robert, ed. Contributions to the Psychobiology of Aging. New York: Springer, 1965.

————, ed. New Thoughts on Old Age. New York: Springer, 1964.

————. "Theories of Human Aging: The Search for a Conceptual Framework," *Journal of Social Issues*, XXI (1965), 13–36.

Kenny, Robert W. "My First Forty Years in California Politics, 1922–1962." Univ. of Calif., Los Angeles, Oral History Program, 1964. Typescript.

Kent, Donald P. "Social and Cultural Factors Influencing the Mental Health of the Aged," *American Journal of Orthopsychiatry*, XXXVI (1966), 680–85.

Kleemeier, Robert W. "Leisure and Disengagement in Retirement," *The Gerontologist*, IV (Dec. 1964), 180–84.

Knepper, Max. "Scrambled Eggs in California," *Current History*, Oct. 1939, pp. 58–60, 64.

Kulp, C. A. "Appraisal of American Provisions for Old-Age Security," *Annals of the American Academy*, CCII (1939), 66–73.

Kutner, Bernard, et al. Five Hundred over Sixty: A Community Survey on Aging. Philadelphia: William F. Fell, 1956.

Kynette vs. California Pension Plan et al. Superior Court, Los Angeles County, file no. 433470.

Lake, Stuart. "If Money," *Saturday Evening Post,* May 11, 1935, pp. 12–13, 121–27.

Lake County Bee (Lakeport, Calif.). For the years 1920–40.

Lane, Robert E. Political Life: Why People Get Involved in Politics. Glencoe, Ill.: Free Press, 1959.

Lansing, E. V., ed. Cowdry's Problems of Aging: Biological and Medical Aspects. Baltimore: Williams and Wilkins, 1952.

Larsen, Charles E. "The EPIC Campaign of 1934," *Pacific Historical Review,* XXVII (1958), 127–47.

Le Brun, Harvey. "Evolution of the American Pension System, 1883–1936," *Sociology and Social Research,* XX (1936), 453–62.

Leuchtenburg, William E. Franklin D. Roosevelt and the New Deal, 1932–1940. New York: Harper, 1963.

Leven, Maurice, et al. America's Capacity to Consume. New York: Review of Reviews, 1934.

Lipset, Seymour Martin. Political Man: The Social Basis of Politics. Garden City, N.Y.: Doubleday, 1960.

Long Beach *Press-Telegram.* For the years 1920–40.

Los Angeles *Daily Journal.* For the years 1920–40.

Los Angeles *Daily News.* For the years 1920–40.

Los Angeles *Evening Herald-Express.* For the years 1920–40.

Los Angeles *Times.* For the years 1920–69.

Lubove, Roy. The Struggle for Social Security, 1900–1935. Cambridge, Mass.: Harvard Univ. Press, 1968.

Ludwig, Edward G., and Robert L. Eichorn. "Age and Disillusionment: A Study of Value Changes Associated with Aging," *Journal of Gerontology,* XXII (1967), 59–65.

Lyon, Charles W. Papers. Univ. of Calif., Los Angeles, Library, Dept. of Special Collections.

McHenry, Dean E. "The Pattern of California Politics," *Western Political Quarterly,* I (1948), 44–53.

McIntosh, Clarence F. "Upton Sinclair and the Epic Movement." Ph.D. diss., Stanford Univ., 1955.

McLain, George. "Old Folks Lobby Report: California State Legislative Action on Social Welfare, 1963 Regular Session." Sacramento, July 15, 1963. Mimeo.

McWilliams, Carey. California: The Great Exception. New York: Current Books, 1949.

———. "Ham and Eggs," *New Republic,* Oct. 25, 1939, pp. 331–33.

———. "Pension Politics in California," *The Nation,* Oct. 1, 1949, pp. 320–22.

———. Southern California Country: An Island on the Land. New York: Duell, Sloan and Pearce, 1946.

Mannheim, Karl. "The Sociological Problem of Generations," in Paul Kecskemeti, ed., Essays on the Sociology of Knowledge (London: Oxford Univ. Press, 1952), pp. 276–322.

Martin, Lillien J., and Clare De Gruchy. Salvaging Old Age. New York: Macmillan, 1930.

Mason, Bruce. "The Townsend Movement," *Southwestern Social Science Quarterly*, XXXV (1954), 36–47.

Maturity. Newsletter of Citizens Advisory Committee on Aging, State of California. For the years 1953–67.

"The Meaning of Ham and Eggs," *New Republic*, Nov. 15, 1939, p. 97.

√Medicare and Social Security Explained. Chicago: Commerce Clearing House, 1965.

Melendy, H. Brett, and Benjamin F. Gilbert. The Governors of California. Georgetown, Calif.: Talisman, 1965.

Mercer, Jane R., and Edgar W. Butler. "Disengagement of the Aged Population and Response Differentials in Survey Research," *Social Forces*, XLVI (1967), 89–96.

Messinger, Sheldon L. "Organizational Transformation: A Case Study of a Declining Social Movement," *American Sociological Review*, XX (1955), 3–10.

Milne, Richard. That Man Townsend. Indianapolis, Ind.: Prosperity, 1935.

Modern Crusader (Long Beach, Calif.). For the years 1934–35.

Moore, Winston and Marian. Out of the Frying Pan. Los Angeles: De Vorss, 1939.

Morgan, James N. "Measuring the Economic Status of the Aged," *International Economic Review*, VI (1965), 1–17.

Nadeau, Remi. Los Angeles: From Mission to Modern City. New York: Longmans, Green, 1960.

Napa *Journal*. For the years 1920–40.

National Ham and Eggs (Los Angeles). For the years 1938–41.

National Townsend Weekly (Los Angeles). For the years 1935–40.

Nelson, Daniel. Unemployed Insurance: The American Experience, 1915–1935. Madison: Univ. of Wis. Press, 1969.

Neuberger, Richard, and Kelley Loe. An Army of the Aged: A History and Analysis of the Townsend Old-Age Pension Plan. Caldwell, Idaho: Caxton, 1936.

New York State Joint Legislative Committee on Problems of the Aging. Birthdays Don't Count. Legislative Document no. 61. 1948.

———. Brightening the Senior Years. Legislative Document no. 81. 1957.

———. Enriching the Years. Legislative Document no. 32. 1953.

New York *Times* (Western ed.). 1963–64.

"Non-Institutional Aged Dependents in San Francisco in Need of Old-Age Pensions," *American Labor Legislation Review*, XVIII (1928), 169–70.

O'Byrne, Arthur Carlyle. "The Political Significance of the Townsend

Movement in California, 1934–1950." M.A. thesis, Univ. of Southern Calif., 1953.

"Old-Age Pension Bill," *American Labor Legislation Review*, XIV (1924), 307–10.

"Old-Age Pensions in California, Massachusetts, New Jersey, and New York in 1935," *Monthly Labor Review*, XLI (1935), 924.

Owen, Russell. "Townsend Talks of His Plans and Hopes," *New York Times Magazine*, Dec. 29, 1935, pp. 3, 15.

Parker, Florence E. "Experience under State Old-Age Pension Acts in 1933," *Monthly Labor Review*, XXXIX (1934), 255–72.

Parsons, Talcott. "Age and Sex in the Social Structure of the United States," in Talcott Parsons, Essays in Sociological Theory (Glencoe, Ill.: Free Press, 1954). Rev. ed., pp. 89–103.

Pasadena *Star-News*. For the years 1920–40.

Patterson, Ellis E. "Reflections of a California Liberal." Univ. of Calif., Los Angeles, Oral History Program, 1965. Typescript.

Peirce, John M. "California's Old-Age Aid," *Tax Digest*, Mar. 1939, pp. 86–91.

Philbrick, Howard R. Legislative Investigative Report. N.p.: Edwin N. Atherton and Associates, 1938.

Philibert, Michel A. "The Emergence of Social Gerontology," *Journal of Social Issues*, XXI (1965), 4–12.

Phillips, Herbert L. Big Wayward Girl: An Informal Political History of California. New York: Doubleday, 1968.

Phillips, John. Inside California: Ten Talks on Subjects of Vital Importance to Every Californian. Los Angeles: Murray and Gee, 1939.

Pinner, Frank, et al. Old Age and Political Behavior: A Case Study. Berkeley: Univ. of Calif. Press, 1959.

"A Place in the Sun," *Time*, Aug. 3, 1962, pp. 46–50.

Pollak, Otto. "Conservatism in Later Maturity and Old Age," *American Sociological Review*, VIII (1943), 175–79.

The Population of California. San Francisco: Commonwealth Club of Calif., 1946.

Preston, Caroline E. "Subjectively Perceived Agedness and Retirement," *Journal of Gerontology*, XXIII (1968), 201–4.

Price, Edward T. "The Future of California's Southland," *Annals of the Association of American Geographers*, Supplement, XLIX (1959), 101–16.

"Public Old-Age Pensions in California, New Jersey, and New York, 1934," *Monthly Labor Review*, XXXIX (1934), 881.

Putnam, Jackson K. "The Influence of the Older Age Groups on California Politics, 1920–1940." Ph.D. diss., Stanford Univ., 1964.

———. "The Persistence of Progressivism in the 1920's: The Case of California," *Pacific Historical Review*, XXXV (1966), 395–411.

Redlands *Daily Facts*. For the years 1920–40.

Rogers, John Walker. The Elder Worker. Commonwealth of Kentucky, Dept. of Labor Bulletin no. 35. Oct. 1929.

Rose, Arnold, and Warren A. Peterson, eds. Older People and Their Social World: The Sub-culture of Aging. Philadelphia: F. A. Davis, 1965.

Roseman, Alvin. "Old-Age Assistance," *Annals of the American Academy,* CCII (1939), 53–59.

Rosenblatt, Aaron. "Interest of Older Persons in Volunteer Activities," *Social Work,* XI (1968), 87–94.

Rosow, Irving. Social Integration of the Aged. New York: Free Press, 1967.

Sacramento *Bee.* For the years 1920–40.

Sacramento *Union.* For the years 1920–40.

San Diego *Sun.* For the years 1920–40.

San Francisco *Chronicle.* For the years 1920–40.

San Gabriel Valley Tribune. For the years 1965–69.

Santa Ana *Register.* For the year 1969.

Santa Cruz *News.* For the years 1920–40.

Santa Rosa *Press-Democrat.* For the years 1920–40.

Schlesinger, Arthur M., Jr. The Politics of Upheaval. Boston: Houghton Mifflin, 1960.

Schmidhauser, John R. "The Political Behavior of Older Persons: A Discussion of Some Frontiers in Research," *Western Political Quarterly,* XI (1958), 113–24.

———. "The Political Influence of the Aged," *The Gerontologist,* VIII (1968), 44–49.

Schramm, Wilbur, and Ruth T. Storey. Little House: A Study of Senior Citizens. Stanford, Calif.: Inst. for Communication Research, Stanford Univ., 1962.

Schramm, Wilbur, and David M. White. "Age, Education, and Economic Status as Factors in Newspaper Reading," in Wilbur Schramm, ed., The Process and Effects of Mass Communication (Urbana: Univ. of Ill. Press, 1954), pp. 71–73.

Senior Californian. Commission on Aging, State of California. For the years 1968–69.

Senior Citizens Sentinel (Los Angeles). For the years 1962–69.

Shock, Nathan W. Trends in Gerontology. 2d ed. Stanford, Calif.: Stanford Univ. Press, 1957.

Sinclair, Upton. The Autobiography of Upton Sinclair. New York: Harcourt, Brace, 1962.

———. The EPIC Plan for California. New York: Farrar, 1934.

———. I, Candidate for Governor, and How I Got Licked. Pasadena, Calif.: Upton Sinclair, 1934.

———. I, Governor of California, and How I Ended Poverty: A True Story of the Future. New York: Farrar & Rinehart, 1933.

Smith, T. Lynn, ed. Problems of America's Aging Population. Gainesville: (Univ. of Fla. Press, 1951).

Smothers, Frank, ed. The States and Their Older Citizens: A Report to the Governors' Conference. Conference of State Governors, Chicago, 1955.

Social Security Unemployment Compensation, Federal and State. Prentice-Hall Looseleaf Reports. Englewood Cliffs, N.J.: Prentice-Hall, 1965–69.

Solomon, Barbara. "Social Functioning of the Economically Dependent Aged," *The Gerontologist*, VII (Sept. 1967), 213–17.

Stewart, Maxwell S. Pensions after Sixty? New York: Public Affairs Committee, 1940.

Stimson, Marshall. Papers. Huntington Library, San Marino, Calif.

Stokes, Randall, and George L. Maddox. "Some Social Factors on Retirement Adaptations," *Journal of Gerontology*, XXII (1967), 329–33.

Stone, Edna L. "Public Old-Age Pensions in the United States," *Monthly Labor Review*, XXII (1926), 1414–22.

The Support of the Aged: A Review of Conditions and Proposals. New York: National Industrial Conference Board, 1931.

"$30 Every Thursday: Analysis of Proposed Life Payments Initiative," *Tax Digest*, Sept. 1938, pp. 311–18.

"Threat of Pension Pressure Groups," *Tax Policy*, Nov. 1939, pp. 1–7.

Thune, Jeanne, et al. "Personality Characteristics of Successful Older Leaders," *Journal of Gerontology*, XXI (1966), 463–70.

Toch, Hans. "Attitudes of the 'Fifty Plus' Age Group: Preliminary Considerations Toward a Longitudinal Survey," *Public Opinion Quarterly*, XVII (1953), 391–94.

Touhy, E. L. "Gerontocracy," *Geriatrics*, V (1950), 337–38.

Townsend, Francis E. New Horizons: An Autobiography. Chicago: J. L. Stewart, 1943.

The Townsend Crusade: An Impartial View of the Townsend Movement and the Probable Effects of the Townsend Plan. New York: Twentieth Century Fund, 1936.

The Townsend Scheme. New York: National Industrial Conference Board, 1936.

United States government publications. All published by the Government Printing Office, Washington, D.C.

[1] Bureau of the Census. Fourteenth Census of the United States, 1920. Vol. II; Vol. IV, "Population, Occupations."

[2] ———. Fifteenth Census of the United States, 1930. "Population," Vol. II; "Population," Vol. III, Pt. I; "Population," Vol. IV, "Occupations."

[3] ———. Sixteenth Census of the United States, 1940. Vol. II, "Characteristics of the Population"; "Population," Vol. II, Pt. I; "Population," Vol. III, "The Labor Force"; "Population," Vol. IV, "Characteristics by Age," Pt. I.

[4] Census Office. Twelfth Census of the United States, 1900. "Population," Vol. I, Pt. I.

[5] Department of Health, Education, and Welfare. Facts on Aging. No. 3. Feb. 1963.

[6] ———. The Nation and Its Older People: A Report of the White House Conference on Aging. 1961.

[7] ———. Selected References on Aging: An Annotated Bibliography. 1959.

[8] Department of Labor, Bureau of Labor Statistics. Care of Aged Persons in the United States. Bulletin no. 489. 1929.

[9] ———. The Cost of American Almshouses. Bulletin no. 386. By Estelle M. Stewart. 1925.

[10] ———. Employment and Economic Status of Older Men and Women. Bulletin no. 1092. 1952.

[11] ———. Public Old-Age Pensions and Insurance in the United States and in Foreign Countries. Bulletin no. 561. 1932.

[12] Federal Emergency Relief Administration. A Selected List of References on Old-Age Security, The United States. No. 3, Pt. I. Comp. by Adelaide R. Hasse. 1935.

[13] Federal Security Agency. The Economic Status of the Aged and Social Programs for Their Support. 1940.

[14] House of Representatives. Old-Age Pensions: Hearings before the Committee on Labor. 73d Cong., 2d sess., 1934.

[15] ———. Old-Age Pension Plans and Organizations: Hearings before the Select Committee Investigating Old-Age Pension Organizations. 74th Cong., 2d sess., 1936.

[16] President's Council on Aging. The Older American. 1963.

[17] Senate. Old-Age and Disability Pensions. Senate Document no. 140. 70th Cong., 1st sess., 1928.

[18] ———. Old-Age Pensions: Hearing before Committee on Pensions. 72d Cong., 1st sess., 1932.

[19] ———, Special Committee on Aging. Economics of Aging: Toward a Full Share in Abundance, A Working Paper. 91st Cong., 1st sess., 1969.

[20] Veterans Administration, Medical and General Reference Library. Care of the Aged: Selected Bibliography. 1950.

Voorhis, Jerry. Confessions of a Congressman. Garden City, N.Y.: Doubleday, 1948.

Walker, Robert A., and Floyd A. Cave. How California Is Governed. New York: Dryden, 1953.

"What Price Old-Age Security?" Transactions (Commonwealth Club of California), XXVII (1933), 337–76.

Whiteman, Luther, and Samuel L. Lewis. Glory Roads: The Psychological State of California. New York: Crowell, 1936.

Witte, Edwin E. Development of the Social Security Act. Madison: Univ. of Wis. Press, 1962.

Workers over 40. New York: National Assn. of Manufacturers, 1938.

Zinberg, Norman E., and Irving Kaufman, eds. Normal Psychology of the Aging Process. New York: International Universities Press. 1963.

Index

Index